BAREFOOT DOCTOR'S
HANDBOOK FOR THE

URBAN
WARRiOR

A SPiRiTUAL SURViVAL GUiDE

BAREFOOT DOCTOR'S HANDBOOK FOR THE

URBAN WARRIOR

A SPIRITUAL SURVIVAL GUIDE

PIATKUS

© 1998 Stephen Russell

First published in 1998 by
Judy Piatkus (Publishers) Ltd
5 Windmill Street, London W1T 2JA
www.piatkus.co.uk

Reprinted 1999, 2000 (three times)

The moral right of the author has been asserted

A catalogue record for this book is available
from the British Library

ISBN 0-7499-1811-X

Edited by Kirsty Fowkes
Designed by the Senate
Illustrations by Roger O'Reilly/Folio

Set in 9.5pt Palatino by
Action Typesetting Ltd, Gloucester

Printed and bound in Great Britain by Biddles Ltd
www.biddles.co.uk

i DEDiCATE THiS BOOK TO WALTER, AND EVERYONE WiTH THE COURAGE TO LOOK BENEATH THE SURFACE AND FiND THEiR OWN WAY THROUGH TO SURViVE, NAY, i SAY THRiVE, ON THiS ROTATiNG LOONY BiN OF A PLANET FOR THE DURATiON, ESPECiALLY THE YOUTH.

CONTENTS

DISCLAIMER
Be warned: what follows is pure propaganda and the author a complete charlatan and fraud.

The information, ideas and suggestions contained in this book are based on a system which is potentially subversive. In essence, it proposes living without morals and returning to your true nature, which it assumes is innocent and free of distortion.

In so doing, your life and, by extension, the lives of those around you can be deeply affected. Whether the effect is positive or negative, helpful or harmful depends entirely upon you, the reader. Though interaction with this Handbook is obviously intended to enhance your experience of reality, the introduction of any catalyst for change in your life is necessarily experimental with unpredictable results. This author therefore takes no responsibility for any outcome arising from your use of the Handbook.

As for this author, while it's certainly true that he's taught the Taoist arts to thousands of people, written a book on the subject, which has so far been read by more than half a million people around the world in twenty languages including Chinese, produced healing trance music which has been enjoyed on every continent, and is health editor of a groovy spiritual lifestyle magazine, it's preposterous, these impressive credentials notwithstanding, that he should have the audacity to set himself up as an expert of this ancient 'system'. As an expert of a system for achieving absolute mastery, he's a fake, being as damaged, confused and unmasterly as the next person.

What he is, in fact, is an artist. An artist with an oblique angle and bizarre tastes, who, in the traditional Taoist mould, for better or for worse, has made his whole life his art-form, his creation, his fully interactive, multi-media, mobile installation and has proceeded to stumble through it like a drunken monkey ever since.

In fact, like any artist, he is no more than a mere interpreter who having adopted the Taoist warrior tradition as his own, worked with it, played with it, danced with it, grabbed and grappled with it for twenty years, has emerged at this point in his travails and deeds of derring do, with one of those humble-but-proud smiles on his face and this book in his hand, proclaiming, 'I have this!'.

This Handbook represents the author's impression (so far) of an ancient system which, though Chinese in origin, is universal in its application and which he now desires, for both altruistic and self-seeking reasons, to share with you, the reader.

So now you know. Suspend your judgement and read on (at your own risk).

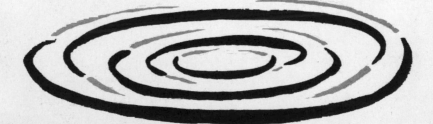

INTRODUCING BAREFOOT DOCTOR AND THE HANDBOOK
Barefoot Doctor here with you, wishing to introduce myself discreetly.

In days of old, throughout the Orient, the barefoot doctor would patrol his local patch, going humbly (barefoot) from village to village, helping the people remain in good spirits and health.

He would do this by administering healing herbs and lotions, acupuncture, massage and energy transfer healing; by teaching martial arts, exercises and meditation techniques; by doing 'miracles' and by playing music on a pippa (lute) or bamboo flute and reciting magical poetry.

His comprehensive healthcare services were offered with the loving heart of a true warrior without concern for financial or personal gain. As reward for his generosity, the local folk would take care of all his needs and ensure he would want for nothing.

This Barefoot Doctor of modern-day Taoist folk-hero fame lives and works (literally barefoot) in accordance with these principles and will never turn someone away who needs healing for having no money.

I see sixty people a week on average, some of whom are too sick to work or, being unemployed, have no money. They bring me flowers, food and even little bits of 'sacred' wood to burn in my fire.

This is not to toot my own horn, I'm as self-centred as the next barefoot doctor. It's just to assure you of my full commitment and integrity in playing the barefoot doctor role to the utmost so that you can simply sit back and enjoy the Handbook without getting jittery.

Though reputed to be somewhat of a rascal in my private life, I have been living as a Taoist urban warrior and experimenting fearlessly with this system for the past twenty years or more, being at the time of writing an old bastard of forty-two, and have taught and been party to the healing of hundreds of thousands of people around the world, directly through my touch and indirectly through my writing, music and broadcasts.

I myself have been taught by some superb 'first generation' teachers, among them R D Laing, Master Han Tao, Sonny Spruce, Nackovitch and F B Kramer, and it is also their work I am humbly continuing in my own way.

This Handbook is part of the result of all that valuable experience and I proffer it now as a full-on gift of love. The relationship you are about to begin with it could constitute a major experiment with your reality.

It is written primarily for your enjoyment, both in the reading and in the after-effect on your life. It contains some pretty heavy stuff and is therefore best treated lightly with a peck of pickled pepper.

Though it happens to contain all the information you need to install the warrior's mind set in your circuitry, the information is presented so as to entertain you and therefore facilitate easy absorption.

This is no mere two-dimensional intellectual explanation (literally a laying out flat on a plain) of a system, but is in fact a total 'sensaround' four-dimensional interactive reading experience.

I am appealing to your true intelligence which lies behind your intellect, the intelligence of your body. Dimension three is introduced by placing the ideas in the context of your 'everyday' life.

Dimension four comes into play during the process of unfoldment you may experience as the information itself unfolds over time.

If you follow the material in sequence, its silken thread will guide you to a full understanding of the Taoist warrior 'system' almost without your realising it's happening.

If you let the book fall open randomly at any page you can use it as a personal oracle or magical counsellor to give you the answer to whichever question is on your mind, to give you a portion of friendly company, a little chuckle and a spot of up-lift to help you on your way.

Focus on whatever's bothering you most at the moment, then once you have read this passage, close your eyes and the Handbook. Now let the Handbook fall open at any page and read that page.

Perhaps it'll give you some elucidation on your situation, perhaps it won't. But may you receive ten thousand benefits from the reading of it.

BACKGROUND VIEW
if you were to look at life on Earth from the point of view of the healer, you'd be forgiven for diagnosing the patient as pretty sick.

It is unnecessary here to enumerate the various ills and stresses affecting our chances of survival on this planet at the present time. No one alive knows whether or not we've passed the point of no return in the process of plundering and polluting our environment; whether the melting of the ice-caps will actually cause our oceans to rise up and flood all sea-level population centres; or if anyone will actually let fire toxic nerve gases in a frenzy of martial one-upmanship during wars which may erupt over water rights. Nobody is sure whether the Hale-Bopp comet was indeed the herald of Armageddon or just another casual celestial body crossing our orbit at 90,000 mph.

Just the other night in London's East End, a young black man was walking along enjoying his freedom to exist, when he was set upon by four young white men who proceeded unprovoked to dowse him with gasoline, set him alight and watch him burn till he died. For him and his family the apocalypse has already come.

More than two thousand years ago, the Hopi 'Indians' prophesied that there would come a time when people would communicate verbally through cobwebs in the sky and build a platform in space. At this time they predicted that life here would be totally nuts. The weather would become erratic, society would become insane, resources would become scarce, the ground would become unstable and the life-giving sun would become our enemy. The conclusion of the prophesy is too dread to mention. Suffice to say that the patient (life on Earth) has arrived at this time in this state and the prognosis isn't so good.

Now you have a choice. You can partially or totally ignore the situation for a short while longer, you can become immobilised with fear, or you can be an urban warrior (or warrioress) and groove on the greatest, most spectacular tragicomic, science-'fiction' drama ever enacted on this planet (probably) until the lights go out. And that's what this Handbook is here to help you do.

Of course, there's always the chance that if enough of us take that path, our combined creative intelligence might forestall things a while and enable us to carry on a little longer in our collective madness.

DEFiNiTiONS
URBAN
Greetings, denizen of the global metropolis!

Since we first started seeing images of Earth taken from space, we have been learning literally to get our minds round the entire planet. We have made exponential advances in communications and computer technology. Alongside this has been a rapid increase of national and international travel which enables us to send ourselves anywhere on the planet with relative ease within twenty-four hours or so.

As a result, there is nothing on Earth, no air, no water, no ground which has not been touched by the poison of our doings. We have generated a vast electronic polluted womb. Its placenta, though disintegrating, is fighting hard

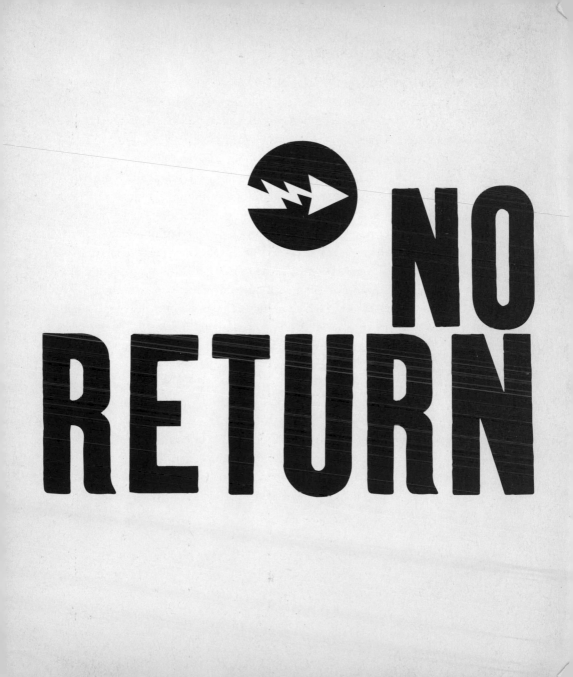

to maintain balance and regenerate itself.

At the same time there is nowhere, not the highest mountain peak, nor the deepest ocean bed, where we cannot or could not remain in contact to share our ideas with each other.

A city is the product of ideas. You have an idea to build a house. You instruct an architect to transform your idea into a more specific idea, who instructs a contractor to transform that into a building, which comprises various components like wiring and plumbing, which themselves are the result of ideas. This building stands in a street which is part of a road system which originated from an idea. You could say that the one cohesive factor in a city, the one thing that makes it a city, is the force of ideas.

You could also say, and I do, that with our communications and transport web, we have created, through the combined force of all our ideas, one huge mother of a global urban sprawl. And you're in it right now. Wherever you may be as you read this, no matter how remote or apparently isolated, you're in it, part of a vast planetary web of population centres linked by planes, cars, boats, phone lines, electric cable, oil pipelines, microwave phones, radio waves, internet, television signals, satellite, postal services and homing pigeons.

You cannot escape. Resistance is futile. The only viable strategy is to accept it and make the most of it by enjoying every moment of it.

Urban is dirty, urban is exciting, urban is dangerous and urban is where opportunity lies, where all your heart's true desires are made manifest if you're willing to risk it.

Take a long slow breath, come back and notice that that's exactly where you are.

WARRIOR

You are an urban warrior.

If you're here reading this book, anywhere in the global urbanised sprawl, dealing with your reality with some degree of consciousness, you're an urban warrior. 'Warrior' may bring to mind all manner of images to you, from the muscle-bound gladiator to the diminutive tai chi master but these are just archetypes. 'Warrior' has the same root as 'war' so when you say you're a warrior it implies that you're at war. This war is an internal one which is taking place in the spiritual realm between the forces of light and the forces of dark throughout the universe and specifically within you.

From the beginning of time the generative, life-affirming current has been at war with the degenerative, entropic, life-negating current and this drama is enacted millennium after millennium by us unwitting puppets.

War is happening in microcosm within each of us and in varying degrees macro-cosmically in our global society and the result to date is the world you see around you.

This is neither a negative nor positive statement but merely a description of a condition.

As a warrior, your challenge is successfully to negotiate this condition in order that you thrive, not just survive, in a state of relaxation and unshakeable, impenetrable wholeness in the very midst of events.

You do this by channelling the forces of light and dark within you into a perpetual dance of equality as opposed to an eternal series of inner street brawls. For this you need all your energy channels open so you can be centred, clear-minded, aware, alert, positive and loving in any conditions in order to appreciate fully and enjoy the miracle of your existence at all times.

When the two opposing forces are in harmony within you the world around you will reflect this and you will manifest harmony wherever you go.

As a warrior you take responsibility for holding the balance between light and dark within you and, by extension, the world around you, and ultimately when you go deep enough, the universe.

It's a big responsibility, the biggest in fact and once you sign on it's irreversible but the pay-off is also the biggest – absolute freedom and a wonderful life for as long as it goes on, of ease, richness, joy and peace in full conscious awareness.

So if you're on for the gambol, say immediately, 'I am an urban warrior. I am willing to take on the responsibility of being a warrior and willing to take on all associated benefits as of now.'

This may seem daft but being a warrior requires you do quite a few daft little rituals just to remind yourself.

TAOISM AND THE TAO
Taoism is a wayward pursuit.

Taoism doesn't exist really. It's not a religion. It's not an institution. It's not even an ism. It's simply an idea, a collection of methods for restoring peace and prolonging life. That's all there is to it. You don't have to believe anything or have blind faith. You don't have to take any oaths. All you have to do is entertain some basic concepts [see next twenty items or so], and practise some easy psycho-physical techniques on a regular basis and you can call yourself a Taoist. Mind you, if you do, do it in a jocular manner because the actual word is a contradiction in terms and is a bit of an in-joke.

Tao roughly translates as 'way', referring to that which happens of itself along the way or Great Thoroughfare of life. This applies as much to the landing of a ladybird upon your summer shirt as it does to the formation of this universe. Underlying and running in the cracks and spaces between reality, the Tao is the primary generative force of existence and, for that matter, non-existence.

Although some overly eager folk over the past few centuries have attempted to institutionalise the idea of Taoism and turn it into a religion of sorts, their attempts have been laughable and have thankfully failed to kill the living spirit of the Tao, unlike other more successful religions. Taoism, the art of living by following only the way that comes naturally, hence wayward, has always appealed to the more individually minded amongst us, which is why, in this epoch of the individual, it is enjoying such a global airing. It originated in ancient China, no one knows how or through whom, but according to legend was passed down by a posse called something like 'The Children of Reflected Light' who were said to be seven feet tall, wear strange clothes and inhabit the high places (mountains). They were said to possess this vast body of knowledge and to disappear without trace once they had passed it on to the locals.

This knowledge trickled down through the millennia, mingling with Buddhism, Confucianism and even Christianity at times, until it reached us today in the form of tai chi, the I Ching, acupuncture and feng shui, to name a few of its better known carriers.

You don't have to renounce any belief or creed you may subscribe to, including gross materialism, to be able to take part in this game. Nor will your involvement in Taoism impinge on anything you hold dear. On the contrary, by following your natural path or Tao you will enhance all existing aspects of your life while adding a few new good'ns into the bargain.

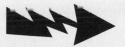

There's only really one of us here looking out from many different faces: name's 'Tao'.

This one central and ubiquitous being sits for eternity in the undifferentiated absolute, doing absolutely nothing. It gets totally bored. Being bored, it grows restless, being restless it grows curious, and so almost without noticing, develops a sense of self, which implies there being something other than self, and the grand, universal game of hide and seek begins. The being begets 'other', which makes two, yin and yang [see *Yin-Yang* p. 14]. Yin-yang proliferates exponentially, as these things do, the ten thousand things come into existence of themselves and you end up with this, the world of appearances.

And thus the Great Being amuses itself by playing this irresistible, inevitable, never-ending game of hide and seek with itself, splitting itself into myriad versions of the original holographic template. Then it pretends to forget it's done that, so that Bob or Joan, Ronald or Snod, Nakovitch or whoever, are now walking around taking themselves seriously as separate, autonomous entities. And that's where the confusion begins, fear and greed are born, wars erupt and so on.

If everyone in the entire universe, every woman, man, centipede, Martian, shark, dog, suicide bomber, saint, butterfly, hooker, bigot, reflexologist and cab-driver, were simultaneously to drop an advanced level, hardcore-heavyweight meditation, and all went deep enough inside, we'd all meet up, along with everyone who's ever lived, ever, in one absurdly mad, huge inner chamber, and to our utter astonishment (feigned of course), we'd, you'd, I'd discover that there'd only been one of us here all the time.

'Tao', pronounced 'dow' and not 'tayo', as I said, means 'way', as in the Japanese version 'do', used for example in 'aikido' – the way of life-force; 'judo' - the gentle way; and 'dodo' – the way of stupidity. Every creature inert and 'ert' has its own individual Tao or path. Every situation has its Tao or way of unfolding. Even every dog has its Tao.

The Tao, however, is not God. God is God, the Tao is the Tao, and words are words. You can't understand the Tao, no one ever could, so don't even bother trying. If you want, you can pray to it, but it will neither listen nor care, so content is it to let things unfold of themselves. However, if you relax and trust the Tao, it will give you everything you need for the rest of your life and beyond.

Just for a metaphysical giggle, pretend for the next seventeen minutes that you are the ultimate entity, then go and drink a cup of tea.

FASCISM
The opposite of Taoism is Fascism.

Taoism essentially means to follow the path of least resistance while always maintaining respect and consideration for the welfare and freedom of all other beings. Fascism means to control the behaviour of others and manipulate them to comply with your particular model of reality, by force if necessary. If you're particularly charismatic or plausible you can gather a following fairly easily because, perversely, many people like to be controlled by someone else. It makes them feel safe and for a while gives the illusion of having no responsibility for their lives. These unfortunates are the anti-warriors.

Fascistic tendencies are to be avoided both in yourself and others as they constrict your energy flow and eventually lead to disease of individuals and entire societies.

Fascists come in many guises, not just in dodgy, erotically suggestive uniforms. Perhaps more alarming are the spiritual fascists, the cultists who believe theirs is the only way. The 'enlightened' masters, mistresses and spiritual leaders, with their entourages of henchmen and hit men, who hypnotise their followers into seeing things their way using fear and threats of excommunication; the healers who tell you to follow only their advice or your life won't work, and the husband who tells his wife she'd be nothing without him; I could go on.

Fascism is following the way of making, ie, forcing, whereas Taoism means following the way of allowing what arises of itself, otherwise known as love.

As an antidote to Fascism, visualise the idea of individual freedom arising from your heart and pouring out of you like a fine vapour which proceeds to envelop everyone on the planet, with double doses for those you consider to exhibit the greatest Fascistic tendencies.

Obviously what they do with it is up to them. If you were even to visualise them responding in a way you think proper it would amount to metaphysical Fascism on your part.

CHI
Life force is crucial to the warrior's existence.

Life force, energy or chi is crucial to the existence of all that lives. Chi is mysterious. You can go your whole life dependent on it without even being aware of its existence. It is ubiquitous. It animates, integrates and pervades everything that exists including spiders. It suffuses the very waters of life. It's probably chi that takes your single socks from the bowels of your washing machine. It provides the intrinsic force necessary in your blood to keep you alive. It is the force of nature that makes the grass grow, the planet turn and the sun burn. It possesses innate intelligence combined with a will to push through. It does not discriminate between 'good' and 'bad' and will animate a deadly virus as readily as the next messiah.

Both the passing by at one million mph of a magnetic cloud 30,000,000 miles wide and the merry prancing of the tiniest quark are impelled by chi. The energy required for you to read and absorb these words is brought to you courtesy of chi. Chi is produced in your body on a daily basis by your internal organs through the assimilation of air, food and drink, and through the impact upon your personal energy field of gravity, light, wind, heat, cold, damp, minerals, chemicals, gases, large objects such as trees and mountains, other people and life-forms, ie, your environment.

You also inherit a finite portion of 'ancestral' chi from your parents at the time of conception, which is stored in your kidneys and serves as a catalyst for the environmental chi.

Chi flows through your body via a complex network of channels or meridians. When its flow is unobstructed you enjoy good health, physically, emotionally and mentally. When its flow is impeded you get sick and when it stops altogether, you die. The most common experience of chi is sexual excitation. This is chi in its 'crude-oil' state.

And this is just the basic model without CD Rom. Using the advanced 'warrior' techniques chi can be harnessed, developed and tuned to such a refined level that it transmutes into 'superhuman' psychic force. You can then use it for a number of important extra-curricular activities. For example, you can create an impenetrable psychic shield for self-defence, self-healing and helping others, be enlightened, be spiritually immortal, perform miracles, make lots of money easily and be an exceptional lover. And all by simply assimilating the information which follows in this Handbook.

If you would like to experience your chi after reading this, sit comfortably and imagine yourself holding an American football-sized object between your palms with the pointed ends facing up and down. Slowly raise and lower the ball about nine times and you'll feel a wooshy sensation in your palms and that's chi.

YIN-YANG
People go, people come, in the dance of equilibrium.

Imagine a multi-media, interactive, electronic, live performance art installation representing the scenario of your existence, as it is right now. There are gadgets and gizmos placed at odd angles, depicting your dreams and schemes, screens flashing images of your memories and fantasies, essence burners giving off familiar smells and aromas, and monitors emitting the sounds of your daily life. The performance aspect comprises you sitting in your deconstructionist armchair, wired, mind and body to the circuitry. As you sit there, various key players in your life walk around the installation and are affected, find it variously, 'moving',' disturbing', and 'fabulous'. The artist has obviously dedicated a lifetime to perfecting the milieu.

This whole installation runs on a special, refined form of electricity called 'chi', which is being produced in a big, solar generator round the back. There is a single, fat, industrial cable running from generator to installation, which houses two separate sub-cables, one conducting a positive charge, the other, a negative. These opposing charges are mutually dependent. One is useless without the other, and so they spend eternity locked into a perpetual dance of equality.

The positive charge is called 'yang', and carries heat which, left unchecked, would cause everything in the installation, including you, to pop, expand, burn and explode.

The negative charge is called 'yin', and carries cold which, unchecked,

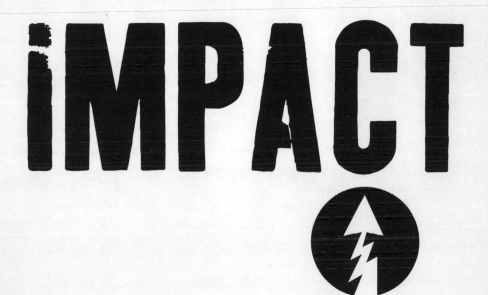

would cause the entire structure including you to shrivel, condense, freeze and implode.

To prevent the installation erupting in flames or collapsing in on itself to form a pile of condensed rubble and congealed bioplasm, it's obviously desirable for these yang and yin charges to be equal in electromotive force, thus ensuring a healthy balance in the ambience of the installation.

Balance, however, is not a static phenomenon. Yin and yang actually move in a complex of alternating currents, so that sometimes there's more yin in the mix and sometimes more yang, depending on time of day, phase of the moon, and season. This produces discernible fluctuations in the status quo.

The lights will start out pleasantly dim, gradually growing dimmer till you can no longer read, at which point they'll start to grow brighter, which will be a relief, until they grow slightly too

bright and your wrinkles start showing. Same with the smells, sounds, climate control, and even your mind, which will go from a whimper to a veritable explosion of ideas, before returning to the void.

In the performance, you don't do anything about this fluctuation; it's there to give a little variation in light and shade. You don't interfere with the process. You don't try to enhance it or alter it in any way. You don't resist it. You simply be aware it's happening and observe which phase the energy's in, small yang, big yang, small yin or big yin, and go with it.

When there's more of the yin and the lights go dim, and it starts getting cold, and you feel like retreating, retreat, ie, stop. When yang's on the rise, and you're feeling restless with heat in your thighs, advance, ie, do something.

Once you start to discern the phase and can feel the yin and yang moving in your life, they become your friends, and their fluctuations level out as evenly as the taste of sweet and sour chicken.

So good night yin and good day yang, yin and yang the life-force gang.

FULL AND EMPTY

The Tao gives and the Tao takes away. When it gives, you're full, when it takes away, you're empty again, ready to be filled with something new. Knowing this won't change your life. The cycle of alternation between yin and yang is inexhaustible. But it may soften the blow of the ebb and the flow.

Yin is empty, yang is full. Yin is soft, yang is hard. Yin comes down, yang goes up. Yin comes in, yang goes out. Yin gets cold, yang heats up. Yin gets damp, yang dries up. Yin is quiet, yang is loud. Yin retreats, yang advances.

Obviously these classifications are merely relative. You cannot have cold without hot, soft without hard, etc. Yin and yang are only meaningful when you compare one phenomenon or phase of activity with another. If, for example, you compare a candle flame to an atomic explosion, both possessing the qualities of light and heat and therefore both presumably yang, the candle would however be considered yin compared to the yang of the explosion.

Yin and yang, like night and day, turn into their opposite number on reaching maximum potential. Thus as the night reaches its darkest moment, the sun is already sending its first tentative rays over the horizon, and those damn birds start their tweeting. As the day reaches its brightest point, the night is already lurking, ready to cover the sky once again. When the passing police siren reaches its loudest moment, the silence is already following in its wake.

It's the same with the energy in your body. If you go to the extremes of physical activity (yang), you exhaust yourself, and have to rest (yin). If you stop for long enough, you grow restless and go back out again for more (yang). Obviously if either yin or yang goes beyond that point, thereby losing its connection with the other, you die. Unchecked yin makes you congeal. Unchecked yang makes you evaporate.

Possibly the most pertinent use of this system of classification is in distinguishing full (yang) from empty (yin) in your relationship with the world. When your energy to go out into the world is strong, ie, yang, and the world appears to receive you, you are considered to be full and the world empty, that is, you go and fill the world. When the world is knocking on your door, and screaming at you from all directions, the world is then full and you'd better be empty!

Often a period of intense outer activity, pressure of work and the social swirl (fullness-yang), will be followed by a period of dullness and nothing happening (emptiness-yin). To fight these fluctuations or in any way resist or pervert the flow of a particular phase, results in distortions in your energy field which lead to disease and eventually death. When the tide comes in, be there to greet it, but don't chase after it when it goes back out.

So when it's dull, let it be dull. It will transform dull into glittering soon enough by itself, as it follows the natural alternation of full and empty. Then when it does glitter again, enjoy it but don't cling to it any more than you would the dullness. That wheel, it keeps a-turning.

TRAiNiNG
The only infallible way is through repetition. The only infallible way is through repetition. The only etc, etc.

Ideally, you get up early enough to give you one clear hour of 'training' time each day. You eagerly leave the residue of the night's dreams among the morning debris of your sleeping pit or sticking like psychic slime to the mesh of your dream-catcher and, having donned your perfectly chosen training kit, layered appropriately for any climatic eventuality, stroll resolutely into your outside training area. Here you do your Taoist warm-up exercise sequence, which completely clears your head, loosens your joints, realigns your spine, stimulates your internal organs, balances your energy and sharpens your focus. You then practise your Taoist fighting forms, shadow boxing sequences which pump up your internal energy a few notches. You finish with meditation exercises and say your warrior's prayer for peace in whatever manner you do that sort of thing.

This puts you in harmony with your surroundings and prepares you to face everyone you'll meet today with equanimity. You bow discreetly and, with your psychic shield reinforced, gird your loins and go and have a shower.

Of course you can substitute this for any form of exercise you like though the Taoist arts of tai chi, hsing i and pakua are among the most effective, efficient and enjoyable. Anything though that will take your attention away from your intellect and into your body will do. Running, walking, rollerblading, swimming, yoga, ballroom dancing, weights, meditation, even mega-advanced super-step aerobics with overdrive – it doesn't really matter as long as you start every day by holding a meeting with yourself where you engage in some sort of intelligent and preferably gentle exercise of mind and/or body before you hold a meeting with anyone else. To do otherwise would be like going out without first 'performing your toilette' – bad form.

It is the repetition of this daily ritual which cumulatively builds your personal power over time. You get good training sessions and crap ones but you do it every day regardless, unless you're feeling poorly, because it's the best drug you've ever found and you're hooked.

Now that's an ideal, and you may feel well off that beam but, if you can inspire yourself to move a few degrees closer towards your own version of that picture, you'll be doing yourself and us a fine service.

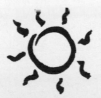

SACRED SPACE

it's good reading this material but unless you designate a short period of your time each day as sacred space for you to touch base with yourself, you stand the risk of your life being just another intellectual conceit.

To operate at all times from the fullness of yourself, as opposed to making use of only a fraction of your potential force, requires that your consciousness inhabits every part of you from the floor up. Your mind must be as much in your hips as it is in your head. If it's only in your head your experience will be merely intellectual and therefore unauthentic.

To be authentic and not just conceptual, your experience must include an awareness of your sacrum. This is the triangular mass of bone between your hip-bones at the base of your spine which, in psycho-physical terms, is the central pole of your being. Sacrum is a Latin word meaning sacred place. It is thus named because it houses your sacred generative energy.

This is most commonly experienced as sexual excitement but also provides the basis for the vitality of your entire psycho-physical structure.

All forms of yogic practice make use of this sacred energy to stimulate the higher psychic centres in your brain for purposes of inner illumination and is the base which supports your entire psychic and physical self. When you are mentally connected from the space between your ears to the space between your hips you are operating from the fullness of yourself. To do this requires that you devote time each day to developing sacral awareness.

Get hip, literally.

Mornings are best, before your mind has time to fall into negative loops and before the world is fully awake, when psychic interference is weakest and the cosmic chi is strongest.

Some people make contact with their sacred self by sitting still and contemplating. Others do it by praying. Others do it during some kind of physical exercise. No matter what kind of touch-base activity you engage in, whether it's tai chi, swimming, walking, yoga, meditation, weights or belly dancing, the important factor is that you do it every day, preferably before you go out to meet your world, and other people, and that you do it with the fullness of yourself.

To make contact with your sacrum, imagine you have a nose there, through which you're breathing in and out. After a few breaths you may start to feel a warm fluid-like sensation there. Keep going and the feeling starts to rise up your spine into your brain. Now that's what it means to be in the fullness of yourself.

SANCTUARY
Give yourself some sanctuary.
It's a scuzzy paradise you find yourself in and there are elements present, demons and hungry ghosts, that will suck your energy. This makes it essential to repair once a day to your own private sanctuary where you can recharge.

You can create a sanctuary in any physical location – a corner of your room, a leafy glade in the park or an entire self-sufficient, eco-efficient mountain hideout, if you can get your hands on one. Place at least one sacred object there, and sacred doesn't mean religious – it can be a toilet brush if that'll serve to remind you – which helps your mind to remember to delineate this as sanctified territory. Candles help to remind you of the miracle of light, and incense pleases the gods and spirits as well as masking the whiff of the mundane.

The words 'sanctuary' and 'sanctify' come from the Latin sanctus meaning holy or whole. Sanctifying a particular spot therefore implies making it holy, as in making it a place where you can experience the wholeness or fullness of yourself, a place to go every day to do your secret touch-base practices, whatever they may be, where you feel protected and safe from interruption.

On entering and leaving make some kind of gesture, a discreet bow of the head for example, to remind yourself that you're dealing with sacred business. Obviously all this is a metaphor for your real sanctuary which is inside you in the inner temple, your centre or tantien [see *The Three Tantiens* p. 41], which is a lot easier to reach if you have access to a space with the right ambience to get you in the mood.

Step in and say out loud 'this is my sacred space' or something equally startling. Then do some of your own secret practice to get you connected to your inner sanctuary. If you're stuck for something to do, there are many fine examples to trigger your imagination in this very Handbook [see Scoopin' the Loop *p. 49 or* Stabilising *p. 115 for example]. This doesn't have to take long – twenty minutes is usually enough to get a satisfactory hit. When you're done, make a contract with yourself to return on a daily basis. When travelling, take the sacred object with you and you can set up temporary sanctuary wherever you are, a bit like the ark of the tabernacle.*

BREATHiNG
Breathing is the most important thing in life. Everything else can wait.

You can go years without human contact, a month without food, a few days without water, but you can't go more than a minute or so without breathing.

That's how important it is.

To appreciate this, hold your breath for 73 seconds. (Do not attempt this if you suffer from respiratory or cardiovascular disorders.)

How you breathe is nearly as crucial as whether you breathe. Breathing acts as a regulator for your entire psycho-physical structure. When you decelerate the tempo of your breathing your mind becomes calmer and your body relaxes more. When you accelerate the tempo your thoughts become more agitated and your body tenses.

Place your hands on your chest just below your ribs. Take a deep breath. Feel something rise and expand? That's your diaphragm, a muscular partition between chest and stomach. When you allow your diaphragm to rise and fall without snagging or halting it, your thoughts and physical energy will flow in a creative direction. When you hold your breath, which you do unconsciously at moments of stress, your thoughts get stuck in a destructive loop and your physical energy falters.

This has nothing to do with learning complex yogic breathing techniques. Simply stop holding your breath and slow the mechanism down.

Your ability to access and channel psychic force depends primarily on your ability to regulate the tempo and smoothness of the movement of your diaphragm. Your ability to attain perpetual inner peace, no matter what the external conditions, depends on your ability to maintain relaxed, natural breath at all times. This can only occur when you pay attention to it.

You may think you haven't time for observing your breath, but it's like driving a car. When you first learn, you have to place all your attention on the mechanics of driving. Later you can pay attention to driving while conducting a conversation with yourself or someone else on entirely unrelated matters. Think of breathing as driving the car. If you don't pay attention you'll crash. Doesn't mean you can't talk or enjoy yourself at the same time.

Throughout the day do random spot checks on your diaphragm. Don't be shy of it, place a warm palm there and think it into relaxing a little more. This procedure will require approximately 15 seconds once you're used to it and is essential because, as a warrior, your life rests on the breath.

As you breathe in and out, you are engaged in an interchange of gases on a global scale.

Every movement of your diaphragm is subtly affecting the atmosphere. It's an activity which brings you into full yet discreet contact with every living creature that breathes on this planet. To optimise on the many personal benefits derived from this process you have to breathe correctly, which involves some basic mechanics.

When you breathe in, your belly must expand and when you breathe out it must contract. Many of us do it in reverse by puffing out the chest and sucking in the belly or abdomen on the in-breath and then collapsing the chest and swelling the abdomen on the out-breath. This works against the natural movement of the diaphragm and reduces the efficiency of your lungs.

Changing this habit now may be tricky, as it will radically alter your experience of life for the better, so if you don't want change stick to incorrect breathing. However, if the prospect of positive change intrigues you, no matter how disruptive it may be temporarily, practise the following visualisation until it becomes automatic. The initial session may last approximately 60 seconds, or as long as it takes to see and feel it. Subsequently it can be performed in the twinkling of an eye. In terms of time spent and life-enhancing payoff, it's a great investment and I strongly suggest you start now.

Imagine you have a sea-sponge in your lower abdomen. It's a special kind of sponge which deals with air instead of water. Picture the sponge in its expanded state filled with air. Now contract the muscles of your lower abdomen, pulling them backwards towards your spine. This movement compresses the sponge and pushes all the air out through your nose or mouth as you exhale. The sponge can now expand on its own as sponges are wont to do, filling with air as you inhale. Squeeze the sponge to breathe out and let it expand on its own to breathe in.

In order to participate you only need to focus on the exhalation as you consciously contract your abdominal muscles, the inhalation occurs all by itself, you need only open to receive the air.

Additionally, your thoughts and energy will flow more peacefully when your breath is inaudible and smooth like a fine round pearl.

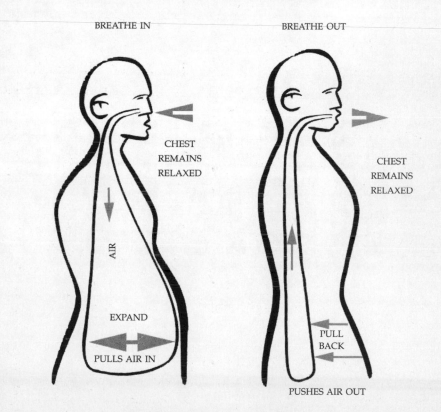

BREATHE IN   BREATHE OUT

CHEST
REMAINS
RELAXED

CHEST
REMAINS
RELAXED

AIR

EXPAND

PULLS AIR IN

PULL
BACK

PUSHES AIR OUT

BREATHING MECHANISM (SIDE VIEW)

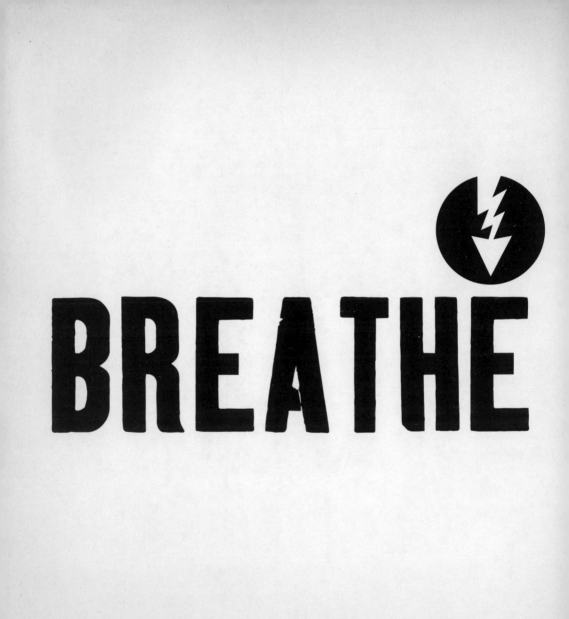

FOUR-STAGE BREATHiNG

Regulating the rhythm of your breath, over time regulates the rhythm of all the events of your life.

The rhythm of your breath directly influences the rhythm of your thoughts and vice versa. When your thoughts slow down, events around you, ie, incoming signals, will eventually slow down to match them, allowing you to accomplish more per second using less energy. Moreover, the rhythm of your breath, a function directly under your control, is the only handle you have on the involuntary rhythm of your heartbeats.

Decelerating your breathing in turn decelerates the essential beat of your heart. Your hard disk is programmed with a preset, finite number of those beats; when that number's up, you die. You might therefore want to consider extending real time for yourself by stretching your portion of beats over a longer period.

Decelerate the tempo of your breath and beat and the pace of life around you will slow down to match yours without any loss on your part.

But to decelerate, you have to remember to focus attention on your breath with frequent regularity during the course of your daily doings. A most simple and effective way to remind yourself is to institute a momentary, almost imperceptible, pause halfway through your in-breath, and again halfway through the out.

Breathing in-in and out-out like this is like tying a piece of ribbon on the little finger of your respiratory system and will help you keep your beats in fine tempo. This four-stage breath method is especially useful when running if you synchronise in-in-out-out with step-step-step-step and will prevent defeat at the hands of breathlessness. It is also handy for walking up steep hills, carrying heavy objects through time and space – passing the occasional piano to a friend, for example – and other such physically demanding situations.

Four-stage breath can also assist you to attain spiritual immortality [see *Scoopin' the Loop* p. 49], so:

Sit back comfortably, maintaining as long a spine as you can [see Posture *p. 31]. Breathe in – pause – in and out – pause – out, nine times, gradually decelerating the tempo as you go. Repeat this procedure often over the next few days and then try it out walking and running, but leave the occasional piano trick for later.*

BODY AWARENESS
Your body, and not just your head, is the field in which you experience everything that happens in your life.

Trouble begins when you spend too much time up in your head. When you do this, energy in your kidneys rises like a hot wind up into your brain. This affects your thought processes, sending your thoughts into loops, and eventually leads to psychic disturbances, headaches, stiff neck, migraine and madness, and generally distorts your reality. Which in reality is happening throughout your body and not just in your head. To develop your chi so you can take full advantage of that reality, you must first gain an awareness of what you're feeling inside your body because that's where chi is produced, stored and accessed. This is the opposite of being conscious of your appearance from the outside, a condition which comes with being up in your head.

The method for developing your chi depends entirely on your being able to send your mind to various parts of your body instantaneously at will. To do this requires that you practise locating areas, say for example your lower abdomen, from inside and feel clearly what's happening there.

After reading this passage, close your eyes and send your mind down from between your ears to an area in your belly just below your navel. Imagine you have a respiration hole (a nose) just below your navel and that you're breathing in and out through it. Become aware of any tension here, of which there's bound to be a little unless you're the Buddha, in which case hope you're enjoying the Handbook but why are you reading it?, and allow it to evaporate as you continue to breathe. After some time, say thirty-six breaths' worth, you may feel a build-up of a sort of heat. (That's chi.) Now repeat this procedure at random points in your body: right palm, left outer knee, solar plexus (stomach), and get so as you can do it faster and faster until it's immediate.

MiNDFULNESS
To normalise, stabilise and harmonise all physical, emotional and mental functions you first have to be aware they're out of balance.

The mindfulness function allows you to monitor what you're doing while you're doing it without interrupting the flow. This allows you to adjust the flow as you go.

It's like watching a character in a movie. She's lying in bed worrying, she's got an uneasy feeling in her stomach, her breathing is shallow, the back of her neck is tense. She's thinking about what she's got to do today, the phone calls she has to make, wondering where she's left her glasses, what will she do if she's lost them, will she be able to take a holiday next month and being aware that her bladder's full. She's so engrossed and entranced in that particular body-mind setup, she's not even aware she's in it. But you're aware she is because you're watching the movie.

Now imagine the movie is interactive. You determine that she's future projecting and click on to bring her mind back to the present moment. You notice her breathing is shallow and click on to deep, regulated breathing. You see her body is locked in a crooked posture so you click on the body uncrumple function. You watch her fear evaporate as her form straightens out and her breathing deepens as she gets out of bed, goes to the bathroom and empties her bladder.

Now imagine that as well as being the person watching that interactive movie, you're also the person in the movie and that you have the ability to watch over and regulate the doings of your own mind and body without getting in the way of the action. That's the mindfulness function, the keys to which will be found in the following sections.

CENTRiNG
Wherever your thought goes, your chi will follow.

Centring is a psycho-physical device for gathering your chi around a single 'point' located one and a quarter inches below your navel [see *The Three Tantiens* p. 41) simply by thinking it there. Once gathered, your chi becomes a unified shape, a hub around which the outside world rotates like the rim of the wheel. Centred thus in the midst of events, your thoughts will be clear enabling you to make clear choices, and your energy will be collected ready to be issued to support those choices.

Your centre lays dormant and inactive until you think it into existence. You do this at first by imagining it to be so and if you keep on imagining it to be so, it will eventually become so. So . . .

Imagine your chi is a pile of extremely valuable gold coins which have been scattered across the floor of your local shopping mall and your centre (below your navel) is a pot. The idea is to gather up all the coins and get them into that pot as swiftly and efficiently as you can before any of the happy shoppers can get there first. And you have to do it with as little fuss as possible to avoid attracting undue attention to the coins. Once you've got all the coins back in the pot, sit back and congratulate yourself: you're rich!

If your chi is scattered like those coins, it will prevent you from being fully present with what you're doing. This means you're leaking chi which is like pissing your life away and should be avoided whenever possible. Centring empowers you, scattering dissipates you. That's all there is to it. Furthermore, by getting good at gathering yourself around your centre through repeated practice, you will instantaneously access your immortal spirit body [see *Spirit Body* p. 57], and enter the 'spiritual' dimension, which will afford you a portion of that grace you're always yearning for and cheer you up like warm broth at the end of a cold, wet day.

So the next time some wise-ass advises you to 'get centred' you'll know what it means even if they don't.

POSTURE
At this precise moment, oh shapeshifter, the physical posture you're adopting is directly affecting your outlook, attitude and disposition.

If you're sitting all crumpled, you'll inhibit your breathing, internal organ function and energy flow, squash your spirit, limit your perception and generally diminish yourself. If, on the other hand, you're expanding to fill the maximum space within your body, both vertically and horizontally, your spirit will sing out in gratitude, your chi will run like the bulls of Pamplona and your entire experience of this sacred moment we're sharing will be enhanced.

Holding yourself in a crumpled posture is like living in a crooked house whose walls are caving in on you. Stress on the building's structure is causing undue pressure on water and waste pipes and, in some places, is causing damage to electrical wiring. Leakage from twisted pipes is causing damp. Cracks in the masonry and gaps around the window and door frames are allowing in draughts and rendering easy access to intruders. If you were living in a house like that you'd either go mental, do a complete restructuring or move.

Your body is your primary environment, your true house. Difference is, you can't move to another one that easily, so that leaves going nuts or shifting shape. The beauty of the shapeshifting choice is that it's easy to do on a moment-by-moment basis, costs nothing, sorts you out immediately and requires no more than an assimilation and frequent conjuring up of the following image:

Your spine is the structural support which holds your skeleton, and therefore the rest of you, vertical. With your breathing gentle and regulated, soften the back of your neck and relax your lower back. Continue to breathe freely and think your spine into lengthening itself. Focus on lengthening from the waist down to the tail bone and from the base of your neck to the crown of your head. At the same time, lengthen up the front of your body from the pubic bone to the top of the breastbone.

Your pelvic girdle and shoulder girdle are the horizontal supports, the joists that enable the structure to house your internal organs while remaining upright without listing or toppling over sideways. While lengthening your structure vertically, simultaneously think your shoulder girdle and pelvic girdle into broadening.

So you're extending your structure's vertical axis both towards the floor and up towards the ceiling, while extending your horizontal axis out to the sides. This affords you maximum space within the available structure in which to play and enhances all psycho-physical functions.

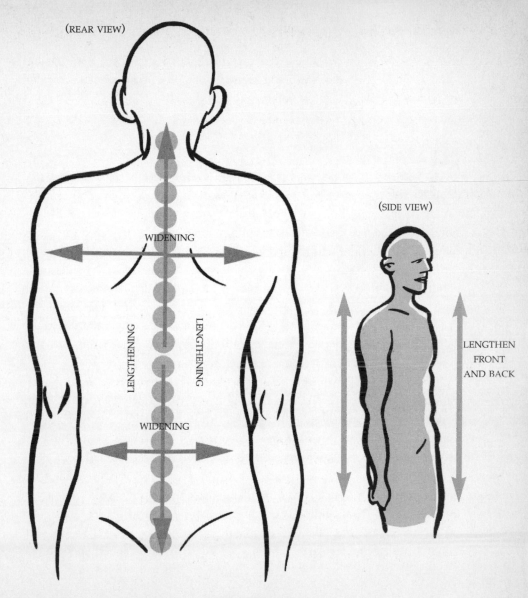

(REAR VIEW)

WIDENING

LENGTHENING   LENGTHENING

WIDENING

(SIDE VIEW)

LENGTHEN
FRONT
AND BACK

POSTURE

Familiarise yourself with this in the static positions first, sitting, standing and lying down, then try it out walking, running, dancing, yoga-ing and any other variation of physical activity you care to partake in.

RELAXATiON

Relaxing does not mean the same as collapsing. You don't have to collapse to relax, but if you don't relax you might have to collapse.

Collapsing is the brother of Crumpled and requires complete inertia. Relaxing, however, is the art of effectively fulfilling the task before you using no more tensile strength and chi than is absolutely necessary. While collapsing seriously limits your range of action, relaxing can be enjoyed while going about your daily doings. Relaxing means to shapeshift in perfect formation with absolute grace like a cheetah on the charge. Relaxing does not mean vegetating while bathing in the gamma rays of your nearest TV set, that's collapsing. Prolonged phases of relaxation deprivation can drop you into extreme involuntary collapse mode which is best avoided.

To do this, stop gripping yourself internally, soften your solar plexus (stomach) region, assume an expansive posture, regulate your breathing, trust your bones to support you and ease off from the thoughts running round in your head. Organise yourself around your centre and expand to fill your physical form. You no longer need to contract and make tension in your body. It won't help you survive. In fact, it will hinder your chances by distorting your shape both physically and mentally, thereby clouding your vision and decision. Relax. Relax all the time, whatever you're doing, however important or trivial. The more challenging the situation, the more you relax. This will make you more effective at everything you do and will attract others who will instinctively wish to bask in the atmosphere you create around you.

If there is one original, universal choice to be made, it's between active relaxation and unnecessary tensing up. When you relax, you automatically desist from distorting the vibrational waves of energy around you, whether incoming or outgoing. Because these waves are endless, they eventually affect the entire universe, however subtly, which is why when you ease off you're doing everyone a service.

The easiest way to explore the difference between these two opposing states so you can decide for yourself which you prefer, is to tense every strand of muscle in your body from your anal sphincters to your eye muscles, and from your little toe muscles to your little finger muscles. Tense them as hard as you can without busting a blood vessel (this is contraindicated if you might be suffering from cardio-vascular or respiratory disease), break the golden rule and hold your breath. Become a totally distorted, tense ghoul like this for nine seconds and then, all of a sudden, as if someone turned the switch off, release.

Repeat this thrice if you want to feel precise. Now R E L A X and luxuriate in the let-go state for a moment or two, and then decide how you want to go from here: ghoul or cool.

SiNKiNG
Drop your fear of sinking, drop everything for a moment and sink.

Sinking is the refinement of relaxing. Sinking means the same as anchoring yourself. Anchoring prevents your mind floating off like a cloud. Floating is beautiful but dangerous if you're not connected to reality, ie, the ground, at the same time, as it makes you top-heavy, easy to topple and gets you taken advantage of.

Sinking is not the same as crumpling in that sinking increases your presence while crumpling reduces it. There is nothing to fear about sinking. The downward pull towards the Earth's centre is counterbalanced by the upward pull of the spirit of vitality [see *Raising the Spirit of Vitality* p. 39]. Grounding yourself in such a dignified (upright) way provides a stable psychic foundation upon which to rest your mind while enabling it to float freely at the same time.

This simultaneous movement of centripetal and centrifugal force [see *Yin-Yang* p. 14] taking place along the length of your spinal column gives you access to the combined power of Heaven and Earth, the power to create with the power to substantiate and is a major factor differentiating you from a slug.

Trusting your bones to hold you upright, let everything else, your flesh, fluids, and energy descend groundwards. This has the effect of rooting you like a tree to the Earth. If you're doing this sitting down, feel the roots reaching through your sitting-bones towards the Earth's centre. If you're standing up, feel the roots going out likewise through the soles of your feet.

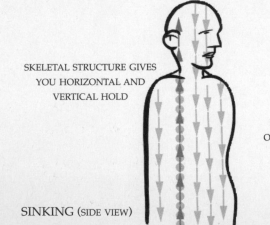

SKELETAL STRUCTURE GIVES
YOU HORIZONTAL AND
VERTICAL HOLD

EVERYTHING ELSE IN AND
ON YOU SINKS EARTHWARDS

SINKING (SIDE VIEW)

YOUR FEET

To stand strong like a warrior in the face of the storm requires you to maintain one pair of strong feet.

Without feet you would lose your ability to stand, walk, run, cycle and balance on high wires as well as other foot-dependent activities you may have taken for granted until now. That's how important they are. So if you're in the fortunate position of being in possession of a pair, now would be a perfect opportunity to go deeper in your relationship with them.

Your feet provide you with a basis for all upright action, supporting you every step of your journey along the Great Thoroughfare.

Keep your attention in your soles next time you're dancing, walking, or running. As well as augmenting the sinking process, this will provide an opportunity for a little shapeshifting groundwork to put you on a firmer footing as you wend your merry way.

Your foot supports you by dint of a highly sophisticated, flexible tripod mechanism, the body's weight ideally dropping through three points: the outside of the heel, the big toe (medial) side of the ball and the little toe (lateral) side of the ball. The extent to which this ground-level mechanism is askew through faulty weight distribution and lazy, fallen arches, is the extent to which your entire physical structure is 'up the pictures'. Following is a little inner footwork to restore balance, add strength and increase stability, both physical and otherwise.

Remove footwear and any Lycra or cotton/mixed fibres that might otherwise be occluding the naked majesty of your feet, ie, be barefoot, and stand comfortably with your feet shoulder-width apart, weight evenly distributed between left and right foot, with the outsides of your feet parallel and facing forwards. With your knees a little bent, your tailbone slightly tucked under so your bum does nay protrude, and your head as if suspended from above by a golden thread, spread your toes as wide as you can, stretching across the balls of your feet. Gently exert an upward pull on the arches (insteps) of your feet and, breathing freely all the while, redistribute your body weight so it's dropping evenly through all three points of the tripod (on both feet).

The daily performance of this feat (average duration, 123 seconds) will, over time, not only improve your general posture but also up your standing in life, metaphorically speaking. Once it has become automatic, which can take anything from three weeks to thirty-three years depending on how much you practise it, how cramped or damaged your feet have been over the years by ill-fitting footwear, and how often you go barefoot, you can try it out walking, running, practising your martial arts, dancing, cycling, wood-chopping, standing in queues, shops and even beauty parlours.

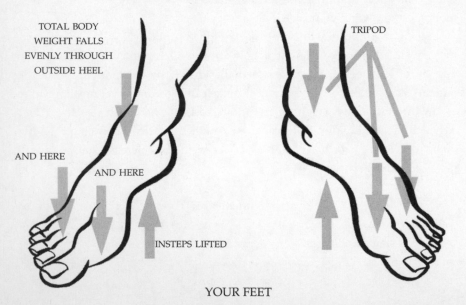

TOTAL BODY
WEIGHT FALLS
EVENLY THROUGH
OUTSIDE HEEL

TRIPOD

AND HERE

AND HERE

INSTEPS LIFTED

YOUR FEET

Although you will probably be using footwear for most of these activities, going barefoot as often as you can, especially on rocky and pebble-strewn terrain is highly recommended for toughening your sole (soul), and for stimulating your general flow of chi through the vital reflex points in the soles.

It also pays to rub, knead and caress them from time to time just to let them know you care. Stop short of buying them fresh-cut flowers but do splash out on some essential oil of lavender, which, if applied between your toes, can prevent fungus and summertime trainers-with-no-socks-on-induced stinkfoot.

RAISING THE SPIRIT OF VITALITY
Keep the energy on top of your head light and sensitive.

If you were to trace a line from the top of your left ear over your head to the top of your right ear, halfway along that line, you'd come to the crown of your head. This is a most mysterious and marvellous part of the universe. It is known by yogis as 'the thousand petalled lotus' and by us Taoists as 'the meeting point of a hundred energies'. It is like an antenna on top of your head which, when connected, gives your brain access to all information (energy) currently available in our cosmos. The only limitations on this are the size of your internal memory, the number of filters you have operating, and speed of your processors to download the information. The Hopis recommend you always keep this point 'open' in order to pick up guidance from higher realms.

That's its external function, but internally it acts as a magnet, drawing your positive, vital energies upwards, literally raising your spirits. It's what gets you out of bed when you could have quite easily whiled away the entire day there and stops you being a bum.

To activate this point, and thereby raise your spirit of vitality to the top of your head, visualise a ball with a diameter of, say, six inches made of sparkling, glittering, special effect-like-light, rotating on its own axis in the air about two inches above your crown. If you practise this until it becomes habitual and automatic, it will keep your mind nimble, active and ready for the main chance.

Alternatively, imagine there is a golden thread attached at one end to the top of your head and at the other to the top of the sky. A gentle upward pull is being exerted on the thread, which has the effect of suspending you from above. This also helps lengthen your spine [see Posture *p. 31].*

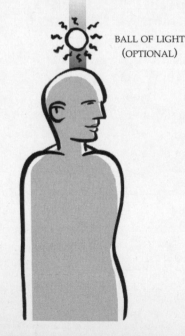

GOLDEN THREAD
SUSPENDS YOUR HEAD

BALL OF LIGHT
(OPTIONAL)

RAISING THE SPIRIT OF VITALITY (SIDE VIEW)

THE THREE TANTiENS
if you're keen to develop an impenetrable, unperturbable core, read this.

Within your physical body there are three psychic power stations or tantiens (fields of heaven), relating to the seven chakras of yoga, which, when acting in unison form your imperishable core and which, with a little extra alchemical jiggery-pokery [see *The Psychic Loop* p. 48], enable you to give birth to your own spirit body [see *Spirit Body* p. 57] which is when that old Taoist magic truly drops, ie kicks in.

The first of these tantiens, the 'ocean of vitality', usually referred to as your centre, is situated one and a quarter inches below your belly button, about two inches back towards your spine. It is responsible for transmuting chi into the physical strength and stamina you need to survive here, as well as providing the necessary sexual urge to prevent you being the last guy. This represents the lowest function of energy, not in a discriminatory way, but in the sense of the basic foundation upon which all life rests.

The next tantien up, the middle one, is called the 'crimson palace' which, as the name implies, is located in the middle of your chest at the level of your heart, about three inches back towards your spine. The crimson palace is responsible for transmuting energy into passion and emotions, without which your life would be as flat and meaningless as an outdated bus pass (unless you need a roach). This is the function that gives you human qualities like love and hate, desire and aversion, generosity and greed, and prevents you from becoming an android.

The uppermost, the 'cave of the original spirit', is situated plumb in the middle of your brain behind your eyes and between your ears roughly where your pineal gland resides. As well as keeping your hard disc in good working order, it is responsible for transmuting energy into intelligence ie assimilating incoming signals from your sense organs and organising them into usable information inside your brain. Also affectionately known as your 'third eye', the upper tantien gives you the ability to see things other eyes can't, a sort of superhuman x-ray vision.

When these three fields of heaven are on and working together, the power to fulfil your heart's desires along with the intelligence to appreciate it will be yours, and what's more you'll be a man (/woman), my son.

Two visualisation and contemplation exercises follow to assist you in accessing this experience.

iNNER LANDSCAPE ViSUALiSATiON

if you're drawn to landscapes, here's a chance to create your own through the technology of 'virtuous' reality.

This is a picture to help you access your three tantiens and thus establish an impenetrable and unperturbable core.

In your lower abdomen is the dark, fathomless, night-time ocean, moonlight reflecting on the waves. The underswell is flowing from front to back inside you. This endless current represents your strength and stamina. Spend some quiet moments synchronising your breathing with the ebb and flow of the waves, then redirect your attention up the face of the cliffs which rise steeply from the sea, along the front of your spinal column into the middle of your chest.

Here you find the crimson palace, perched in all its splendour at the cliff top, doors and windows open wide to emit a strong crimson light for all within a thousand miles to see. This light represents your inexhaustible love and passion for life. Spend a while synchronising your breathing with the outpouring of those crimson rays, then start your ascent up the mountainside passing the jade pagoda (your cervical vertebrae/neck) until you finally reach the cave of the original spirit, nestled in the

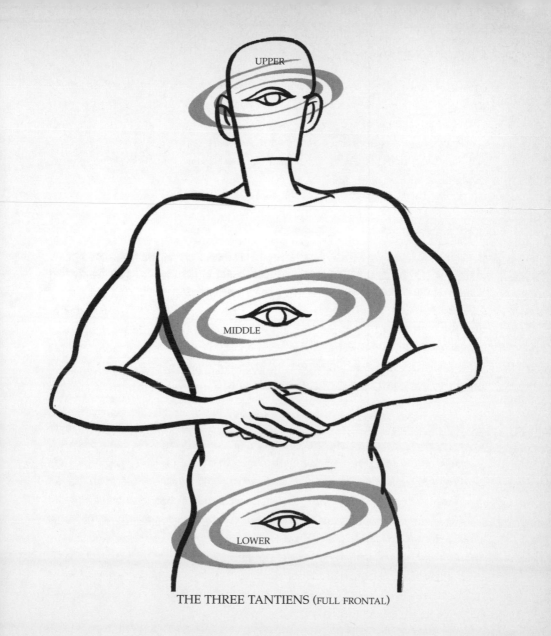

THE THREE TANTIENS (FULL FRONTAL)

rarefied air of the highest mountain peaks which pierce the sky just below the crown of your head. Here you sit, uplit in crimson, sidelit in other-worldly, whitish original spirit light, the sound of crashing waves far below you, looking out into infinite inner space. This endless space represents the infinite intelligence which is yours when you send in three inner landscape visualisation packet tops, and answer this simple question: 'Who are you, really?'

THE THREE FRIENDLY DEITIES VISUALISATION

if you've ever found the Father, Son and Holy Ghost scenario a little too daunting and distant to see you through the occasional dark night of the soul, here's a trinity that will warm the cockles of your belly and brain as well as your heart.

In introducing this unlikeliest of holy Taoist trinities, Watchful Fox, Benefactor and the Phat Controller, friendly deities three, I feel obliged to warn you that integration of the following visualisation into your repertoire may put the kind of eccentricity into your practice that can qualify you for fully-fledged membership of the IWT (Institute of Wayward Taoism).

In the cave of the original spirit lives a character called Watchful Fox. As the name would imply, he is sharp, sly and cunning and doesn't miss a trick. He has acute powers of observation and notices absolutely everything. He's genetically programmed that way – foxes didn't survive as one of the most successful species of urban warrior by dozing. Picture him now, sitting secretively inside your head, alert to the slightest change and poised for immediate action. WF represents your faculty of impartial intelligence, made possible by the function of your uppermost tantien. As you focus on him, contemplate the quality of eternal duration.

In the crimson palace, seated regally on the main throne in the main throne room, is Benefactor, literally Doer Of Good Deeds, who radiates kindness and unconditional

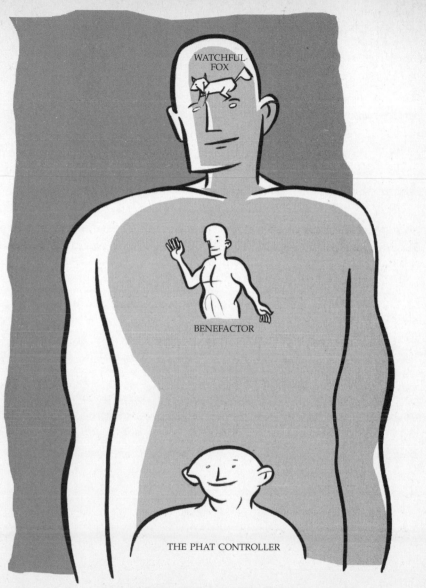

THE THREE FRIENDLY DEITIES (FRONT VIEW)

love for the benefit of your good self and everyone else you'll ever encounter. That's his job: to warm up your experience of reality by giving you that feeling of peaceful contentment you often crave which results from a healthy through-flow of love between you and others. When spending time with him, contemplate the quality of absolute harmony.

Meanwhile, way down the cliffside, deep in your lower abdomen, at his usual table in the restaurant he frequents along that most prime and salubrious portion of sea-front real-estate, sits the Phat Controller. PC is a sturdy, stalwart fellow, the fat buddha type, who takes command of every situation, whispering so that others have to strain to hear his down-to-earth brand of wisdom. Don-like and calmly centred in his bearing and demeanour, he is happy to lead from behind or below, so to speak. When you're moving with the Phat Controller, contemplate the quality of limitless power.

If this particular visualisation does appeal, make a point of meeting up with the friendly deities three often enough that you can hold a clear picture of all three at the same time, each sitting in his particular domain. This will effectively open and balance the psychic forces appertaining to your three tantiens. Naturally these characters are 'merely' personifications of those forces, so feel perfectly free to change names and genders (theirs) if you should so choose. Also, if inclined towards that sort of thing, you can call on them individually or severally as staunch allies in times of need [see *Club Culture* p. 132].

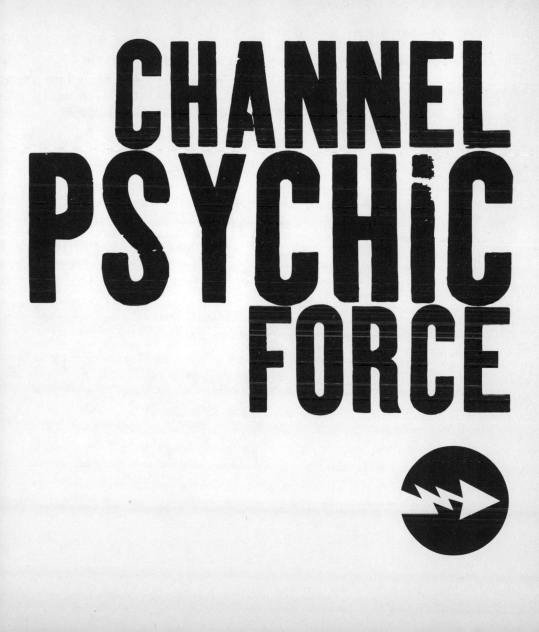

THE PSYCHiC LOOP

There is a primordial energy loop within your body, even as we speak, in which other-worldly psychic force has been circulating since before you were born and will be after you've hung up your Earth-boots for good. Tapping into this inner flow will affect your life in profound ways so leave this alone if you want to keep things like they are (as if that were possible!).

Your body runs on a system of twelve major and seventy-two minor arteries, invisible to the naked eye, which carry chi to and fro between your vital organs. In addition to these are a group of eight 'extra' arteries, psychic ISDN lines, capable of conducting the more potent, prenatal variety of psychic force usually found developed to a high degree in warriors, sorcerers, gurus and other assorted types of spiritual masters and mistresses. Of these psychic arteries, two – the Control and Functionality channels – are of supreme importance. Control regulates the entire flow of yang [see *Yin-Yang* p. 14] chi in your body which, among other things, gives you the ability to ideate (entertain ideas), while Functionality regulates the flow of yin, which, among other things, gives you power to make those ideas functional.

Together they have potential to form a continuous loop around which you can send your psychic force in perpetual yin-yang orbit. This purifies, intensifies and accelerates your flow of psychic force, enabling you within about ninety days of regular practice to delineate the shape of your own spirit body [see *Spirit Body* p. 57]. This is crucial for anyone interested in attaining spiritual immortality and the lesser spiritual feats of physical longevity, astral travel, being invisible, and doing general miracles of healing and treasure materialisation. [Items on these and other skills associated with psychic loop work appear later in this Handbook.] Control begins right between your legs (in more ways than one), runs like a string of fine pearls up the back of your spine, over the crown of your head and down through the back of your face, where it merges with Functionality. Functionality then runs down the back of your throat, through the front of your body, behind your pubic bone, past the root of your genitalia to merge with Control right between your legs once again.

This loop is activated through the following exercise which combines visualisation and breathing.

SCOOPIN' THE LOOP
When you feel your spirit droop, run and scoop the cosmic loop.
Having familiarised yourself with the above idea, and the four-stage breathing method, organise a tranquil moment and sit quietly, free from external distraction. After grokking (absorbing the information with your whole being, not just your intellect) the following passage, close your eyes, and . . .

Picture your own personal cosmic loop running up along the rear of your backbone, from your tailbone to the top of your head and down through the front, behind your pubic bone, and back up again. As you breathe in, imagine the air rising up your control channel from tailbone to crown, and as you breathe out, imagine it dropping through your functionality channel from crown to genitals.

To help harness your mind to your breath, introduce the four-stage breathing method, dropping the pauses in halfway up the ascent and halfway down the descent.

Train yourself to complete nine rounds with full conscious awareness with an eased off attitude and happy disposition and, within no more than nine sittings, the loop'll be scoopin' automatically and continuously whenever you care to check in on it.

As soon as this becomes apparent, scoop your cosmic loop while running, walking, standing, talking, dancing, tai chi-ing, yoga-ing, fornicating, sitting in departure lounges, suburban lounges and leisure lounges, waiting in traffic jams (get a bicycle), cycling and, in short, during every imaginable act.

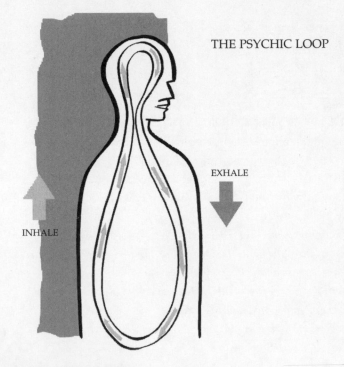

THE PSYCHIC LOOP

EXHALE

INHALE

SLiNGiNG iT ALL TOGETHER

i can fool you no longer on the subject of your current metaphysical situation. Just reading what i have to say about it is no longer going to be enough.

In moving to a deeper level of training, wherein the powers of extrasensory perception, advanced mood management and many other assorted bonuses will be bestowed upon you, it will presently be necessary for you to review everything, from *Training* through to *The Psychic Loop*. Proceeding otherwise is only recommended for those with a penchant for gaps.

The following activity, if partaken of fully, will at first tie up all your mental capacity, probably in a nice knot, subsequently releasing it reinforced with renewed clarity and vigour. Taking time at this stage to sling together all the information thus far presented during the course of a single sitting (approximately one half hour) will afford you access to the dimension or context in which your spirit body, whose faint outline you may even now be starting to discern, spends its days and nights while you go gallivanting. Regular access to this realm will stabilise your psychic structure that necessary extra portion to make it safe for you to practise the psychic shield, cloak of invisibility and astral travel techniques among others, mentioned later in this Handbook.

Having refamiliarised yourself with the basic building blocks: breathing, posture, centring, relaxing, sinking, etc, bring them all into play, one by one, as you complete nine slow breath cycles focusing on your three tantiens. The picture will probably move in and out of focus, but with practice it'll get easier to hold steady. Now, holding your three tantiens firmly in the frame, introduce the psychic loop, running vertically around them. Using four-stage breathing, scoop your psychic loop nine times with full conscious awareness.

Without becoming obsessive about it, practise this during dedicated time every day for about nine and a half weeks, throwing in the odd impromptu flash-on-flash off, mobile mini-session during the course of your daily doings. This will strengthen and protect your spirit body so you can take it out to play with all the other fallen angels without it getting mucky wings.

PSYCHIC SHIELDING
HORIZONTAL HOOP

Once you've learned to scoop the loop, do the psychic hula-hoop.

There is a belt of psychic force rotating in a clockwise direction around you on the horizontal plane at 186,000 miles per second (speed of light), at the level of your lower tantien at an average distance of approximately six feet from your body. It is like the rim of a wheel with a twelve-foot diameter, whose hub is located just in front of your spine, one and a half inches below your navel, rapidly spinning around you like a supercharged psychic Hawaiian hula-hoop. It remains in the latent state until activated by your mind, at which point it provides a protective psychic force shield capable of deflecting any harmful or violent energy aimed at your person, whether by thought, word or deed.

You set it in motion simply by visualising it. This requires belief in the power of your imagination but, over time with regular visualisation, you will be able to feel its immense gyroscopic force surrounding you. Once set spinning, it pretty much remains in a state of perpetual motion, and will only require the occasional maintenance (visualisation) session to adjust the angle of spin or correct any glitches that may result from ordinary distortions in your energy field.

Sit comfortably and picture a belt of psychic force rotating like the rings of Saturn around your waist at 186,000 miles per second in a clockwise direction (left to right). The material of the belt itself is composed of an infinite quantity of special effects light particles, each particle itself spinning at 186,000 miles per second around its own individual axis. Looking down at the belt in full spin, you see that this wheel of light is actually solid all the way from hub to circumference. Maintaining your centre and posture, and using four-stage breathing and scoopin' the loop, keep your awareness on

HORIZONTAL LOOP (FRONT VIEW)

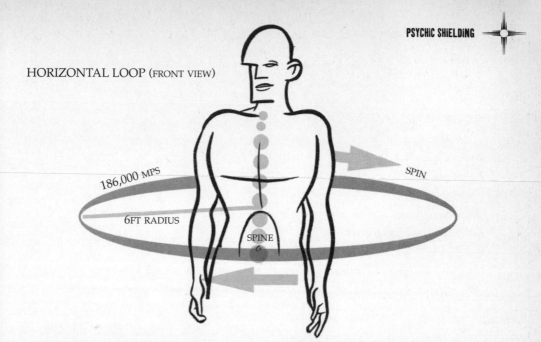

186,000 MPS

SPIN

6FT RADIUS

SPINE

the spin for about seventeen minutes or until you can take the tingling in your tantien not a moment longer, become dizzy or simply grow bored.

When pernicious energy of any kind, psychic, physical or viral, attempts to invade your person, it will be spun off in whichever direction you choose by using your intention [see *Intention* p. 64]. You can also use it to clear a space around you when you require more dancing room in a crowded club, for example.

You're sitting idling outside the cafe on the canal eating a sandwich. It's a weekday. Everyone's at work and the loch is deserted. Out of the silence, a rumpus erupts from the direction of the black sheds to your left. Although you can't see them, it sounds like a couple of drunks shouting and kicking cans around. Suddenly, out of the shadows emerges a young man, maybe nineteen or twenty and built absurdly huge. Blinking in the light, he fixes his bloodshot eye on you and comes stumbling directly towards you, grunting and snorting like an intoxicated bull, tattered clothes caked in vomit, and the filth of a thousand nations liberally smeared on all available fleshy surfaces and under fingernails, piling up in heavier concentrations around his numerous visible sores, cuts and abrasions.

'Eiiurrh!' you exclaim, biting into your sandwich, as you contemplate the health risks of physical contact or being vomited upon. At this point, the psychic hoop you've been visualising from time to time in your inner training sessions instantaneously activates itself before your very eyes.

He continues to approach you, stare fixed with blood-poisoned intent but, when he reaches a distance of about six feet from your person, exactly where you see the hoop spinning, he is spun off in another direction as if someone was operating him by remote control.

You make a wish for his recovery, marvel at the effectiveness of your psychic hula hoop and, with an attitude of gratitude, continue about your business.

PSYCHIC EGG
Instead of fighting with arm and leg, climb inside your psychic egg.

See yourself in a giant egg composed of special effects particles of solid light, each spinning on its own axis at 186,000 miles per second. Like a cosmic Humpty Dumpty you are surrounded front, back, sides overhead and underfoot by its intense, though invisible-to-the-naked-eye radiance.

The nucleus of this egg is in your lower tantien below your navel. This nucleus also acts as the hub of a wheel, whose rim forms your psychic loop, a belt of energy rotating on the horizontal plane at the level of your waist, around the

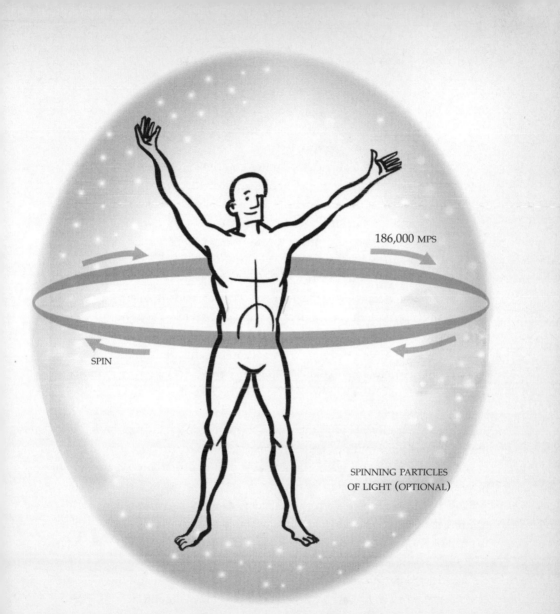

186,000 MPS

SPIN

SPINNING PARTICLES
OF LIGHT (OPTIONAL)

PSYCHIC EGG (FRONT VIEW)

'equator' of the egg. This egg acts like a giant psychic membrane which, like a psychic sunblock, filters out all harmful rays emitted by other people. In theory, it can also protect you from malaria carrying mosquitoes and airborne viruses, though there is not a scrap of medical evidence to support this.

The egg remains in latent state until you activate it with visualisation power. Once activated, it provides an effective shield against psychic attack. Remember all forms of attack begin as attack thoughts, ie, psychically. Even a basic thug attack on the street begins with attack words, which themselves arise from attack thoughts, unless of course you're involved in gangster business or open warfare, in which case they usually skip the words and cut to the chase.

Whenever someone, a jilted lover for example, sends life-negating wishes in your direction, you may consider this a psychic attack. Thoughts always hit their target, like heat-guided missiles, that's how voodoo works. It's the same when someone's jealous of you. Negative thoughts directed at you will impact on your energy field and do damage to your person. In your upper tantien in the centre of your brain, you have psychic radar facilities which enable you to pick up incoming psychic missiles but, because you cannot keep your attention paranoidly fixed on the radar screen all day and night, what with having a life to live and all, the people in design have provided you with the psychic shield facility to ward off all attack, willy nilly, at any time of day or night, regardless of your state of mind.

The best way to deal with the shield is to visualise it in your morning training session, and then give it the quick once-over from time to time during the rest of your waking hours, ending with another more in-depth look in just before going to sleep.

As well as offering you protection from psychic, physical and possibly viral attack, the egg also has psychic beacon and psychic magnet functions (though only with extra practice).

The beacon function allows you to radiate psycho-spiritual 'light' in public places, thus enhancing both your own charisma and the harmonious vibrations in your immediate environment.

The magnet function allows you to draw positive energy towards you. This energy can come in many forms including money, love and other assorted happy surprises.

It is strongly recommended by the Institute of Wayward Taoism that you include this visualisation in your daily routine and use it before setting off on all cycling expeditions through busy city centres.

Remember that without regular practice of this visualisation, along with such basics as scoopin' the loop, your egg may become scrambled.

SPiRiT BODY
What follows could be purely fictional unless you believe It's true, at which point it could feasibly transform itself into fact (now that's magic).

Like the Tao, from which all phenomena arise, your spirit body goes on for ever. Your metaphysical hard disk drive bearing the information from all your various existences and container for your own individual brand of pure consciousness started out before the birth of Father Time and will continue long after his demise. When you were attracted to the mating of your own mother and father at your conception on that propitious day so long ago, it was your spirit body, carrying with it all the trace memories of your former and future existences, which delivered you there safely on implantation and stayed with you throughout your gestation period. As you took your first breath, it retreated from the harsh glare of local reality into that invisible, silent realm where spirit bodies reside. When you hang up your Earth boots it will be there (wherever that is) to carry you on to the next meta-adventure. It doesn't share your local values about right and wrong or pleasant and painful, and will lead you willy nilly to whichever lesson you need next to assist you in the process of your healthy growth.

If you can connect with your spirit body in full conscious awareness while in your present physical shape, you will be in the privileged position of having a considerable chunk of voting power with regard to your own fate. Spiritual masters and mistresses, senior warriors who have this ability, can not only determine the hour and atmosphere of their own death (and I'm not referring to the folly of suicide), but also determine which celestial sphere they wish to bliss out in from there on. Of course, this ability also confers upon the bearer the power to determine the nature and outcome of all upcoming events and situations on the local plane while still possessed of the mortal coil, as well as the ability to see clearly into past and future at will.

Furthermore, in this capacity as sorcerer ie one who is connected to Source (not HP), the accomplished warrior can perform miracles of healing and treasure materialisation, become invisible, be surrounded in a protective psychic shield, walk in perpetual peace, and even enjoy a better standard of sex [see *Sex* p. 164].

Regular performance of the exercise given in *Slinging It All Together* p. 50, will provide the link you need to make contact with your spirit body, but you can speed the process by doing the following visualisation with some regularity, which will acquaint you with it in graphic style.

Nestled in the space between your belly button and centre of your chest is a small being (sb) created in your likeness in all ways but one: no flaws. Perfect from head to toe, from core to iddy-biddy aura, sb veritably glows with the refined light of absolute perfection. As you breathe slowly in and out, imagine your breath is a pump which is inflating sb until your entire physical form is filled with it. This process of inflation continues until sb expands beyond the so-called borders of your body, at which point you notice sb has become SB (spirit body). As you continue to pump and watch, SB presses on with its rapid expansion programme, attaining the size of a large family house, and ever onwards and outwards until, cutting a long story short, the entire known universe is contained in your spirit body.

In this state of omnicontinence and therefore presumably omnipresence, omniscience and omnipotence, you consider having the universe renamed something a little less hackneyed, can come up with no instant improvement, and fumble awhile in the deep freeze of your ancient memory for the reason you chose to expand like this in the first place. Something springs to mind, and after a minute's defrosting in the microwave, you remember. Becoming aware of all you contain, you bestow blessings of divine love on all that is, just like you'd expect a being of this magnitude to do for you. When you've had enough of this heady task, start using your breath as a reverse pump to deflate SB down to manageable day-to-day size inside you, and slowly return to local reality.

Point is, next time you're praying for protection, riding your bicycle through busy city streets, or are strapped into your seat on a turbulent transatlantic night-flight, you may like to consider that the recipient of that prayer could actually be none other than your own SB.

EASING OFF
Ease off!

You want something. Could be anything: to party in Polynesia for twenty-three days, to project your immortal spirit body beyond the ninth celestial sphere and ride the winds of the western sky on the back of a golden dragon, to record a CD of tunes, to tidy your drawers, carouse with your lover, amass a large treasure, negotiate a deal, cook lobster thermadore, whatever.

Having clearly decided to proceed with manifesting your desire [see *Intention* p. 64], you have a choice to make: click on 'difficult' if you want the process to involve effort and hardship, click on 'easy ' if you feel you deserve things to come your way of themselves, naturally and effortlessly?

Though the same amount of work or personal application will be required for either choice, 'difficult' will drain your resources, tire you and limit your enjoyment of both process and result, while 'easy' will allow you space to appreciate the wonders of your existence as the object of your choice sails serenely within reach of your gracious grasp.

The word effort ('e'= out, 'fort' = strength) means putting strength out to get something. When effort is exerted, reserve strength is called upon to supplement the subsequent insufficiency. This places strain on your vital organs which suddenly have to work extra hard just to maintain the internal status quo. When your vital organs get strained, your mood deteriorates and your perception dulls and distorts. This makes the process of getting what you want a drag on your chi, and when your chi drags the whole world drags with you so souring the fruits of your labour. It'll rain in Polynesia, your tunes won't swing, there'll be moths in your draws, and the lobster thermadore will lay on your chest.

Obviously there's a bias to my thrust towards the easy tip because, as any good warrior knows, if you want something to come to you easily, ease off; use only as much energy as you need for the task at hand. If it still isn't coming easily, then ease off some more.

Easing off is not synonymous with slacking [see *Procrastination vs Idling* p. 79], and in no way implies being ineffectual. On the contrary, when you contain rather than splurge your chi in pursuit of a goal, your vital organs will be more relaxed and energy efficient, thereby preserving chi to support you in your work. You will then emit a friendly vibration which will attract rather than repel the objects of your desire. This is a case of less is more.

Consider how the child's balloon travels further when you tap it lightly with focused intention, than when you wallop it with force. Let your chi be that balloon as you tap it towards the object of your desire, and no more huffing and puffing for you, my esteemed reader.

Use any of the following affirmations [see *Affirmation* p. 133] frequently for a couple of days:

I need no longer struggle and strain to get what I want. There's nothing heroic about the busted gut or tensed jaw, these are pastimes for fools. I deserve to have things be easy for me, this doesn't make me lazy. I'm willing to ease off on myself now and let things come to me. I ease off on the world now and, as I do, the world eases off on me – now there's more space for us all to play in. I choose 'easy' so everything is easy for me.

And especially:

I am not a slacker, I'm just choosing ease, for I am free to take things as easy as I please.

INVESTING IN LOSS
if you want your Tao to deliver the best, invest in loss because more is less.

The orthodox slant on investment policy is only invest to make gains. The way of the contemporary urban warrior, by contrast, is to invest in loss. This is not to suggest the warrior is a sucker. Simply that, rather than invest your energy for a return in momentary gain, you invest in decreasing your self-image.

The more you increase your self-image, ie, the myth of who you are, what you do, what you own and what you want, the more unwieldy you become. By carrying that psycho-emotional junk in your travelling trunk, you lose mobility, flexibility and adaptability, and therefore freedom.

When you invest in loss of the myth of who you are, you reduce the load, thereby reducing wind-drag coefficient. This makes it easier for you to move freely from adventure to adventure and increases your chances of being in the right place at the right time for reality to work its full quota of magic on your behalf.

So, rather than expending vast sums of mental energy gripping on to all the elements that comprise your life-story, release your grip and let the Tao take the strain. When you allow the story to unfold on its own, thereby containing your energy, you can respond more effectively as events occur (like CNN news).

Visualise yourself as a pure, radiant being, with no baggage from the past or plans for the future.

What follows is the 'nobody' contemplation. It requires courage to perform as it constitutes an experiment with reality, playing with your sense of identity as it does.

THE NOBODY CONTEMPLATiON

Look around you or simply think of all you own, are paying off for, or renting, in other words, all your 'possessions'. Make a list if you like and say to yourself,' 'I am not these possessions' as in 'I am not this house, I am not this telephone, I am not this rubber biscuit', etc.

Now think of everything you desire and aspire to and say, 'I am not my desires and aspirations' as in ' I am not that different house, I am not that personal satellite phone with built-in modem, fax and organiser, I am not that chocolate oliver', etc.

And on to all those who people your friendly world, and especially the ones you care for most: think of them all (though you should do this in a fairly abstract way to avoid spending too long and losing the plot), and say, 'I am not these people' as in 'I am not Phi Phi the perfect woman, I am not Joio Ktoojaw the perfect man, I am not my mother, I am not my son, I'm not really anyone', etc.

Now think of all your habits and addictions, your weekly visit to the acupuncturist, the way you throw your towel on the bathroom floor, the reefers you don't inhale, and say, 'I am not my habits or addictions', etc.

Think of your aversions, allergies and phobias, and say , 'I am not these aversions, allergies or phobias' as in 'I am not this phobia about getting caught in a locked laundromat with a three-toed sloth', etc.

Finally, think of your body, with all its bits and pieces: energy, nerves, blood, assorted fluids, aches, pains, bones, organs, flesh, outer appearance, and say, 'I am not my body'.

Feel it. You're not your possessions, your desires, your people, your habits, your fears, you're not even your body. You're simply nobody. Revel in the freedom of it, then move out on to the street, a busy, grimy street preferably, and be nobody, absolutely no one at all. Being no one at all, you've nothing to lose, you're just atoms moving in the everything, child of the Tao, and everything is yours.

This is an exercise in making the ultimate investment, investment in loss of all to gain all. Practising it at those times when the story of your life is getting too ponderous to transport easily will yield feelings of great relief and free-spiritedness.

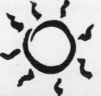

iNTENTiON

Everything you do requires you first be clear about what kind of outcome you intend.

Stop and examine your intention as regards this page. Do you want to read it to amuse yourself, distract yourself, stretch yourself, or simply as a momentary companion to chum you along through the odd lonely bedtime, breakfast or colonic irrigation session?

As soon as your intention is clear, read on. When you arrive at the last word on the page, stop again and notice whether the experience of reading had the desired effect. If so, this will have demonstrated how clear intention produces clear results. If not, it could mean that the intervening passage between here and the last word is just so much tosh, but you won't know that until you've read the page.

Whenever you undertake something, however big or small, you must first have a clear intention as to the desired outcome, not in detail, but in essence. Take the example of wanting to finish this page. First you ascertain that you intend to get to the last word within the next three minutes, feeling refreshed and illuminated on the subject of intention. You see this as a picture or short series of frames, portraying you and the finished page, projected up on to your 'intention screen' which hangs on the wall on the inside of your forehead where you can watch it comfortably from your vantage point in the cave of your original spirit (the pineal gland in the middle of your brain). Next you feel it as an impulse in your crimson palace (the heart centre in the middle of your chest), a desire to finish the page. Lastly you experience a discreet surge of vital power arising in your ocean of chi (in your lower abdomen), which gives you the strength to move your eyes while holding your attention on the meaning of the text.

And before you know it, as is the way with these things, you've arrived here at the end of the page, with only enough time to hear that when you're not clear with yourself about your intentions, you'll send unclear messages to others, who will become confused in your presence, and together you'll add to the general confusion. If, though, as a warrior, you prefer to reduce the level of general confusion in your world, you must start with clarifying your intention with yourself. Or at least intend to.

Being able to focus your intention and harness it to the passion in your heart and chi in your belly, generates a force as real as diamonds. Ultimately, your choice of intention in any situation, however serious or otherwise, is between creating harmony or discord.

And the last word is 'tosh'. Or is it?

REAL STRENGTH
Real strength, the superhuman kind that warriors like, comes from a unity of intention, passion and energy.

You have the intention to carry that heavy garbage bag down three flights of stairs to put out in the street. It's been in the narrow hallway now for too long and every time you've tripped over it, you've built up more of a passion to move it. The message moves down from your brain (upper tantien) where you've conceptualised the action, into your chest (middle tantien), where you feel desire for that action to occur, and then into your belly (lower tantien), where your chi (energy) is finally mobilised and the result is one more bulging black bin liner festooning the street.

If all three are not working in unison, your actions will be unfocused and that bulging black bin liner will be stinking out the hallway for another day.

This applies to any movement, however big or small. For you to be fully effective in any situation, there must be a unity of mind, emotion and follow-through. So, before lifting your next heavy object – that piano for example –

pause for a moment. Clarify your intention to move it to the other side of the room. See it clearly in its new position by the fireplace on the 'intention screen' in the centre of your brain. Feel the desire in your chest to move it. Finally, access the chi in your belly that will give you the follow-through to do so. You can apply this in the face of any challenge that crops up along the way. Your creative projects in general, though hopefully being more far-reaching than garbage removal and piano relocation, nevertheless depend for their success on your utilisation of this same force of unified strength. It's all well and good my having the intention to write this Handbook, for instance, as well as having the passion to do so, but without the energy to follow through, I could no more finish it and hand it in to the publisher on disc compatible with their technology along with two hard copies of the manuscript, on time, than I could lift that piano.

Say I had the intention and the follow-through but not the passion, I might complete it, but what I'd have in my hand when I walked in to the publishers, proclaiming 'I have this!', would be a dry and lifeless affair, and I doubt you'd be reading it now.

A deficiency of any of the three components of true strength: intention, passion, energy, will result in a deficiency of success at the project's end, whether it be successfully buttering your toast, or successfully campaigning to clear the roads of fossil-fuel-burning combustion engines.

To develop unified strength, practise scoopin' the loop and slinging it all together on a daily basis for at least eighty-one days, and may none of your creative endeavours be success-deficient ever again.

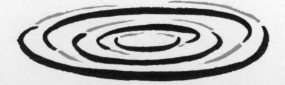

SOFTNESS
True strength derives from softness.

It is a misconception that true strength is hard. Hard is inflexible and eventually causes rigidity, resulting in impaired use of the musculo-skeletal system. This is false strength.

It's the difference between being an oak and a willow. You may think of the oak in all its mightiness as the more steadfast of the two, but when that hurricane comes, the flexible, lithe Ms Willow will bend and yield to the oncoming force, thereby maintaining her roots and preserving her life, while rigid old Mr Oak will snap and topple like a lollipop.

Let softness be your motto. Let your touch be soft. Let your thoughts be soft. Let your words be soft. Let your movements be soft. This does not make you a softy. Softness does not mean jelly-like. It's the same as the difference between relaxing and collapsing. You maintain the firmness and integrity of your imperishable core at all times while allowing your mind and body to remain soft and supple. Your thoughts will then lose all jagged edges and your movements will appear boneless, ie, flowing and graceful.

In your middle tantien, the crimson palace in the centre of your chest, there is a vial containing precious vapour of softness. You open the vial and watch as the vapour escapes. Watch it circulate and radiate like a fine coloured mist all around your body, bones, organs, blood, fluids, brain, nerves, tendons, ligaments, muscles, connective tissue and all. Feel it softening you all over until you feel fully bathed, then let it radiate outwards through your chest until the whole world's immersed in it.

Now focus on the indestructible strength gathered in your lower tantien and spine, and just sit there for a while being strong in softness.

This is another way of saying 'Relax, sink, and ease off!'

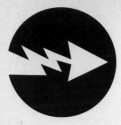

EASY

MEDITATION

Meditate on your life, that is, let your whole life be your meditation.

A group of uptown, spiritual disciples, 'doing meditation', sitting in full lotus, index fingers and thumbs forming circles, basking in the sanctimonious after-silence of their big-up, weekly omming session, may not actually be meditating at all. Thinking of pay rises, new lovers, school fees and hairstyles, they may as well be doing line dancing.

Meditating does not mean 'doing meditation' as in versions of the above, it simply means paying attention. Whatever you're doing, whether counting your breaths or counting your winnings at the one-arm bandit (fruit) machine, that's where you place your full attention. The under-age graffiti artist in the throes of 'writing' is probably more in a state of pure meditation than those meditators at their weekly meeting (no reference to any actual persons, living or dead, intended).

Paying attention to what you're doing requires you be still inside while the outside world moves all around you. This requires practise at everything we've discussed so far which is best done, initially, sitting still without distraction. Once you've got the picture set square in the frame, however, with benefit of full horizontal and vertical hold, take it outside and play with it. Meditate walking down the street, sitting in traffic jams (get a bicycle), in bars, washing dishes, sitting at the computer, in short, while you work, rest and play. This will increase your alertness and enable you to see into the heart of what's going on around you.

The advanced urban warrior could be walking down the street, centred and still in the midst of external events, be set upon by a gang of unscrupulous villains, ward off their attack using the psychic shield technique, and continue merrily waywards without a flicker of disturbance in the meditation process. Now that's meditation!

Sitting comfortably, doing nothing, empty your mind and do nothing. It's as simple as that.

However, if you need extra help in remembering sometimes, try counting. Count everything: your breath, your footsteps, the ringing tone on the telephone; or do the 'deer exercise', which involves squeezing and relaxing your anal sphincter and pelvic floor muscles at about 60 beats per minute (one squeeze and relax cycle per second).

Count up to nine, say, and start again. Then you can count multiples of nine and so on. Doesn't matter if you lose count, the tax people will never find out, it's simply a method of tying up your monkey mind so you're free to pay attention to what's really going on.

OBSERVATION VS JUDGEMENT

Draw your awareness back towards the centre of your brain, the upper tantien into the cave of your original spirit, and work towards keeping it there all the time, whatever the weather, for the rest of your life.

When you do this with your eyes closed, gaze softly into the screen hanging on the wall behind your forehead. When the screen is not in use, ie, no thoughts are arising, it displays scenes of endless inner space, selected from your randomiser. When, however, your thoughts kick in, fractal-like images appear on the screen in kaleidoscopic array complete with portions of chaos factor.

As these images appear, you simply observe them. You don't bother to judge them: 'That's a nice one, I think I'll keep it', or, 'I don't like that one, throw it out!'. You just watch impartially. They're only shapes after all. Nor do you judge yourself for entertaining such images. They're just images. For example, you see an image of yourself betraying your friend. Don't judge yourself as a traitor, it's just an image. Be loving towards yourself and allow your mind to throw up all the images of depravity or magnificence it wants. Acting out is a different story.

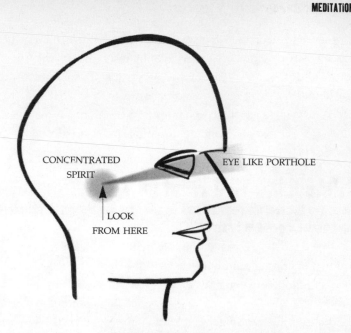

CONCENTRATED
SPIRIT

EYE LIKE PORTHOLE

LOOK
FROM HERE

MEDITATION

After a while (on a good day), these mental apparitions seem to subside, leaving your mind clear and free to respond naturally to whatever's happening as it's happening, without wasting energy on unnecessary mental meanderings.

When you do this with your eyes open, it makes no difference. Your eyes are just the bifocal camera lens. The 'outside world' images you're 'seeing' are merely more shapes and patterns projected on to your inner screen. As you watch the screen with gentle gaze, images will appear of people, cars, dogs, buildings, mountain lions, whatever. Simply watch with loving impartiality from the comfort of your own cave, judging no one lest ye be judged yourself.

Not judging, however, does not mean not discriminating. Someone approaches you on the street, dirt of one thousand years coating every surface, smelling strongly of faeces, urine, vomit and beer, and threatens to French-kiss you. You don't go, 'It's just an image, it's just a smell, this is just revulsion in my stomach, I love you unconditionally, please touch your tongue to mine.' No. You say, 'It's just an image, it's just a smell, this is just revulsion, I'm outa here!' That's how you combine impartial observation with discrimination.

STRADDLiNG TWO WORLDS AT ONCE

There are two worlds running side by side, the visible world and the invisible world. The warrior's game is to straddle both at once.

As above, so below, as within, so without, etc, means that there are two realities operating simultaneously in the same 'physical space', even as we speak. Right before you now, there is the world you can see and the world you can't.

The invisible world generates and supports the visible world from within, pushing outwards from the nucleus of every atom of every being. The visible world is like a cover thrown over the invisible world, not only to keep out the wet and dirt, but also to stop it being seen. Otherwise the game of hide and seek would be over too soon and we'd have to find something else to do with eternity.

Just like your computer, the entire illusion runs on ones and zeros, ons and offs.

The visible world is 'on' and the invisible world is 'off'. You can't get 'on' without 'off' and vice versa [see *Yin-Yang* p. 14]. The Tao [see *Taoism and the Tao* p. 8] could be described in a limited fashion as oscillating between the two faster than 186,000 miles per second (speed of light).

The invisible world contains all the information that ever existed or ever will exist. In that world there is no time, no past, no future, just one present moment that's going on and on and on, like a washing machine eternally held on that notch on the dial just before the water gurgles in. The invisible world is the realm of your spirit body [see *Spirit Body* p. 57].

What you're dealing with in this warrior business is a crisscross between two worlds. You're practising bringing your spirit body out to play in the local world, while training your local self to feel at home on the other side. In so doing, you're 'spiritualising' the local world to facilitate your magical operations and miracle workings, while familiarising your local, mortal self with life on the other side. This not only makes your final crossing less of a deal, but also helps you maintain perspective while still on this side.

The invisible realm is where prayers go and where guidance, protection, providence and healing come from. It's where your spirit, in company of all other spirits, sits for eternity, watching as you go through lifetime after lifetime, dream after dream. Nothing changes there. The eternal moment remains for ever in place on the unchanging face of your G-Shock timepiece. Here (there) in the realm of absolute reality, the supreme ultimate, tai chi wonderland, will be found the heavenly elixir which confers spirit body immortality. You go there to recharge at source, you return enriched in vision and power. This enables you to continue on the path to your full unfoldment, while helping others along the way.

It is through oscillating between visible and invisible realms that you develop psychic power and are able to foretell the future or see someone's past in a passing cloud formation, spread of tarot cards or hexagrams of the I Ching. Access to this realm is within you. There's no big, secret door behind a rock near a stone circle, by an ancient pyramid in the mountainous jungles of Peru. The door is inside each and every one of us. It can be opened by scoopin' the loop and slinging it all together. The idea is to open that door, climb in, and stay there for the duration of your time on Earth, while going about your daily urban warrior existence. In so doing, you're effectively straddling both worlds, thus being in it but not of it, and hence invested of the super-sensory sensibilities and powers commensurate with that privileged position. This enables you to do deeds on the local plane that contribute to the well-being and contentment of your fellow time-travellers, while simultaneously having a party.

The visible, outer world of form and appearance, the arena and stage upon which we collectively play out the human drama is a metaphor for the invisible, inner realm. Thus we physically conduct formalised rituals in the visible realm to represent otherwise inexplicable metaphysical processes occurring in the invisible realm. The purpose of ceremonial magic, including that practised by official religions and other occult organisations, is to remind us to access the door to the invisible realm within, through whichever method suits, and which in this Handbook comprises the wayward Taoist approach to life, death and everything in-between.

LETTiNG GO
'So what!', you may well exclaim, on reading all these words. So what indeed.

You sit there alone in a state of mild agitation, the primordial monster of encroaching insanity threatening to escape through the cracks in the plasterboard of the reality you constructed so neatly, and engulf you in its slimy, entropic discharge. Your plans seem to have gone awry and you're racked with doubts about the choices you made that got you into this position in the first place. Who did you think you were anyway, thinking you could take destiny into your own hands like that?

So you're disappointed. So what! Disappointment's only disappointment.

It will be transmuted into its opposite by the immutable law of yin and yang anyway.

So, so what. May sound impolite or downright uncompassionate, but really, so what.

The thing about 'so what' is that it's got an edge, a small portion of anger released every time you say it. That's its advantage over 'never mind', which is also good and valid, but only when you truly don't mind. Most of the time, though, especially when the disappointment's just recently dropped, you do mind. So with that faint hint of churlish delinquency, stand up, release that irritation and boldly proclaim, 'So what!'

So when you experience frustration, disappointment and self-doubt, as your brilliantly conceived plans go astray and leave you stranded, try a 'so what' session for yourself.

One by one, think of the things about your life that are pissing you off or causing you undue stress and drop a 'so what': 'but I'll lose my job – so what!; but Charlene/Charley will leave me – so what!; but I'll die – so what!'. That's it, be brutal, gently brutal, until you've cleansed yourself of all attachments, and then you can sit down and call yourself the buddha.

Note: it is contraindicated to say, 'so what,' to someone else if they tell you of their travails and suffering. First, they might not understand your sense of humour and secondly, it's for them to say for themselves, so don't deprive them of that pleasure.

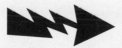

DISTINGUISHING FULL FROM EMPTY

As any singer or athlete knows, if you want to get a lungful of air, you first have to exhale fully. By the same principle, if you want to get a full day of satisfying life, you must empty yourself, mind, heart, bowels and, to some extent, even wallet, on a daily basis.

Meanwhile, you're addicted to fullness, fullness of mind, fullness of heart, fullness of belly, and fullness of pocket. You like to fill your mind with thoughts (fantasies and projections), yours and other people's, as when you watch TV or read books (Handbooks, for example); you fill your heart with desire (for love); you fill your belly with food, and your pockets with money (on a good day). If, however, you were to empty your mind of thoughts, your heart of desire, your belly of food, and your pockets of money, not only would you be a hungry, penniless boddhisatva (enlightened being on the way to full buddhahood status), but you would also be creating a vacuum. According to the law of yang and yin (full and empty), vacuums will always be filled. In fact, fullness (abundance) cannot enter anything but an empty space (receptacle).

By emptying your mind of thoughts, you make space for new
information, realisations, visions and dreams.
By emptying your heart of desires, you make space for peace and quiet
compassion.
By emptying your belly of food, you make room for chi.
By emptying your pockets of money (give some away to someone who
needs it more) you make room for riches.

The courage required to be empty merely depends on trusting the immutable law of yin and yang: what's empty will become full, what's full will become empty. So if it's fullness you crave, a life filled with everything you want, seek emptiness instead. (This is an example of investing in loss.) The following visualisation will help you into emptiness.

Draw your mind back into the cave of the original spirit and imagine a flat LED computer screen hanging on the wall behind your forehead. There's an icon for every thought currently in your mind. Use your mouse and drag them one by one into the trash. When you've emptied your desktop, go into special menu and click on 'empty trash'. This will not erase your hard disk's memory, or in any other way impair normal thinking processes.

Meanwhile, down in your chest, see your heart like one of those free-standing Edwardian baths filled with unruly desires instead of warm water, and simply pull the plug out. Watch until the final drop of desire has drained away and let it fill up with compassion instead.

As for your belly, visualise yourself enjoying a good bowel movement and afterwards let the chi in your lower tantien make you feel warm and safe.

Finally, concerning your pockets, let them not bulge. Give some money away every day and otherwise carry only as much as you need and no more. This will reduce some harmful effects of mugging and give you somewhere to put your hands when you feel self-conscious.

FEAR OF THE VOID

Running away from the void thinking it was death, one day, you stumbled into the void by chance and found a new way to spend your day.

Fear of being empty (minded, hearted, stomached or pocketed), originally arises from fear of the void, ie, death. Tempting you to avoid the void is what the advertising industry makes its living from. Think of all the chocolate, alcohol, tobacco, sex, drugs, CDs, cups of tea, shopping expeditions for unnecessary consumer goods, TV programmes, long nights out in club and restaurant and meaningless conversations that have been had in order to avoid the void.

But, as you know, the void is your natural habitat, your place of origin before that sperm implanted and this endless round of shopping kicked in. Like the depths of the ocean from which life sprang, the void gave birth to all existence. There is nothing, literally nothing, to fear there.

On the contrary, daily bathing in its mysterious waters is to immerse yourself in the pool of youth, truth, good looks and vitality. Scuba diving in it is to submerge yourself in the depths of eternal consciousness and life itself.

This is another way of saying, 'invest in loss'.

After reading this, close your eyes and withdraw your consciousness into the cave of original spirit in the centre of your brain. Imagine yourself sitting like a little buddha in your cave, nestled high among the mountain peaks of the 'Enlightenment' range. Standing up, you walk to the cave mouth and stand on the ledge at the edge of the precipice of the void. Before you, above you, below you, behind you (after you've made your way over to the other side of the mountains) and to the sides of you, there is nothing except the endless void. So you gird your loins, steel your courage and do the expected thing: you jump.

Free-falling thus in the void, you're surprised to notice that you feel safe and exhilarated at the same time, as if you were floating in the womb of the 'great mother' herself. Relaxing into this primordial state, everything in your world falls into clear perspective, it finally rains up and down the length of the land, there's clean water to drink again, and the crops grow abundantly.

Voiding your mind on a regular basis, like the regular voiding of bladder or bowel, is crucial for full functionality of the system. Just like the physical variety of voiding, psychic voiding sessions can be long or short, depending on mood and time available. Thus in the course of a busy day (or night), a short, eighty-one second motion will suffice to stave off mental flatulence and constipation, and keep encroaching madness at bay. Obviously, when you've got time and the fancy grabs you, it's perfectly safe and acceptable to take the newspaper and stay in there for the rest of the day if you want.

IDLING VS PROCRASTINATION
idling is part of moving with the natural flow of your life, procrastination is when you're blocking it. That doesn't necessarily mean it's bad for you, though.

When you're idling you're following the natural progression from a phase of action (yang) to a phase of rest (yin). This is moving with the flow and is good for your health as it gives you a chance to recharge. When you're procrastinating you're blocking that progression by stalling unnaturally in the yin. Disrupting the flow like this causes a build-up of pressure in the system, which causes leaks and unnecessary energy drainage.

Idling is like pulling over to the side of the road on a hot day for a rest, parking and letting the engine quietly tick over in neutral to keep the air-conditioning going while all the other trucks and cars speed past.

Procrastination is like stalling in the middle of the street and causing a traffic jam. (Suicide, the extreme version of procrastination, is like turning off your engine and throwing the keys away.)

Idling time is essential for the busy urban warrior. Idling is a way of releasing into the flow or Tao.

Simply letting your thoughts drift. If you like the pictures, watch them, if you don't, change them. Entertaining the odd fantasy or two, relishing a pleasant memory, gloating over a well-sprung plan. Starting to become aware of your breath, you slow it down, relaxing and sinking, perhaps scoopin' some loop, sending your spirit body out on a marvellous adventure, or simply whispering sweet nothings in the ear of your favourite deity.

So kick back and enter the idle zone, drop into the void, and let your mind go on holiday whenever you get the chance. It is through sojourns in the psychic chillin' lounge such as these, that the likes of Einstein, Picasso, Photek, and Nakovitch, not to mention Lao Tse and Divine Crushing Fist, were able to receive the inspiration for the contributions they made.

Procrastination, like constipation, on the other hand, is a way of holding on and holding up the flow of inspiration. While idler's face is bold and beatific, procrastinator's is cowardly and turgid. Procrastination, like when you 'try' to tidy the room instead of tidying it, or when the members of the men's group spend the session discussing what they're going to discuss instead of discussing it, is a complete fear-ridden waste of time, and you'd have been better off staying home and having an early night. Procrastination can usually be spotted as it creeps up behind you. The tell-tale signs are thinking about one thing while doing another, nervous disposition possibly accompanied by nail-biting, cuticle-picking, mouth-wall chewing, cigarette smoking, tea drinking, pacing up and down and scowling, and a distracted look in the eye. Procrastination is often associated with anxiety, inappropriate masturbation and self-loathing.

Sometimes it seems to occur of itself unavoidably like an extra-terrestrial attack from Procrastinus, god of gridlock. At these times, take note of the signs. If your general tone of experience is negative and unpleasant and you suspect an attack, let the pressure build until you can takes that slacking no more and, turning that energy to your advantage, gird your loins and proclaim out loud, 'I am willing to risk my entire future on my next move!', which is no risk really, because without your next move, whatever it is, you won't have a future. Then get up and do something different (see ya's laters).

You can also affirm [see Affirmations *p. 133], 'The more I idle, the more I achieve. My idling sessions are filled with bliss and eastern promise', or, 'I use my procrastination sessions for building up a counter charge to catapult me back into the current.'*

So when, fine warrior, the path before you appears obstructed and you feel stuck and inert, don't indulge in procrastination or masturbation for too long, instead take some time for recreation, to idle and literally recreate yourself as the author of this fine conundrum [see *Authorship* below] and ease yourself into the next chapter of your own personal story.

AUTHORSHiP
Remember, it's you who wrote the story of your life. No one or nothing else could have written it for you, they wouldn't have had the time.

Long ago, before the illusion of linear time began for you, when you were still an immortal spirit unfettered by physical form, living in eternal present moment awareness, you got restless one day, hopped into the future and wrote a treatment for your life story in retrospect. You took it to the powers that be, gathered the necessary support, were put in touch with your mum and dad and, before you knew it, were lying there screaming as they changed your diapers. But don't let that memory of being a helpless bairn fool you. You wrote this story exactly as it is and, no matter how rough you've made it look at times, you've done an amazing job. You've literally placed yourself in a maze.

Possibly tosh, nevertheless, as a model for conjecture it's as valid as any other. So let's assume for the sake of experimentation that it's accurate and look at what it implies.

Being the author of your own life story literally gives you authority over your life. This means you can no longer be a victim of other people or circumstances because you wrote it exactly the way it's happening for you; they didn't. It means you've even chosen the moment and manner of your own death and that there's no grim reaper except in your imagination.

Taking on this ultimate responsibility as author is a huge step in claiming your own power as a warrior and will lend authenticity to your life. It should also be taken lightly, however, with a pinch of salt, because being too intense about it can lead to confusion, megalomania or paranoia.

Visualise your spirit sitting like a big buddha in the centre of the field of time writing the story of your life from the heart of this big, fat, present moment, where past and future meet. For the part of the story beginning now, write an adventure full of everything you want and include a magnificent finale.

Literally write the story down as you'd like it to go and see what happens.

There is an acupoint at the top of your forehead in the middle which, when stimulated, gives you the sensation of being in the lateral time-field and in control of your own destiny. Press your forefinger into it lightly for a minute or so for a short, lateral reality hit.

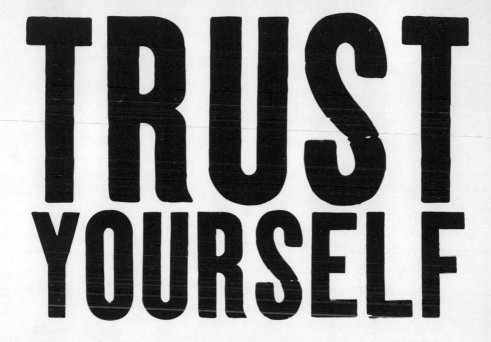

TRUST YOURSELF

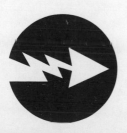

TRUST

Trust is a basic warrior requirement. Without it you're wasting valuable time and energy.

Trust isn't a concept in your mind, it's a feeling in your belly, your tantien.

You go for a helicopter ride and you're a little nervous. It's your first time and before you climb in you look up at the main propeller and pray it stays attached and keeps turning. You wonder if the mechanics have tightened all the screws. Taking off you feel a noticeable adrenalin surge. Now your little metal bubble is flying at full altitude and there's nothing left to do but sit there.

Every few moments you wonder about the propeller and the tightness of the screws and whether the pilot knows what she's doing. Your body tenses but there's nothing you can do to change the situation and you want to enjoy this ride, so you relax your breathing and let your body soften a little. You decide to trust the floor to hold you up and to trust the pilot not to have an epileptic fit. Above all, you decide to trust yourself in having chosen this adventure and you have a top time.

On the other hand you could have decided to remain tense and untrusting and when you got back safe though sickly and staggered out, you'd have wondered why you hadn't let go and enjoyed it, but alas too late.

Obviously this is a metaphor for your life. Relax and trust it or stay tense and waste it. It's probably all predetermined anyway so stop your being such a scaredy cat and say 'I trust myself.'

TRUST YOURSELF
Don't trust this book, don't trust me, trust yourself.

You get taught as a child that you can't trust anyone. And that's partially true. You can't trust anyone to behave in a specific way to suit you. That's not trust anyway, but expectation.

You can trust everyone to be human, with all the quirks and inconsistencies us humans display, including disloyalty, dishonesty, and downright treachery. We are all capable of the entire range of human behaviour, given the circumstances, from absolute saintliness to abject depravity. Trusting someone to limit their sphere of action to one narrow band on the spectrum is idealistic and will inevitably lead to disappointment.

On the other hand, you can decide to trust that everyone is doing their best according to their particular stage of development, and to give everyone their appropriate berth. For this to work you have to trust yourself to make and have made the right choices that will lead you on the path to your healthy growth. You have to trust yourself to come through every experience safely and enriched. But don't trust what I'm saying. Listen and then decide for yourself. Does this information sit easily in your belly? If so then maybe I've given you enough indicators for you to trust yourself around me. It's not a matter of whether you trust me or not.

Trusting yourself requires that you exercise your power of discrimination, which arises from deep within your belly. You know when you trust yourself around someone because your belly feels settled and your heart feels warm. When you're with someone or in a situation where your chest feels tight and you have a nagging sense of unease in your gut and you've gone through the relaxing, sinking and centring procedure, established it's not a stomach bug and still you've got that negative feeling, then get away from there, and don't waste any time about it.

A nice altered state can be achieved by saying 'I trust myself' over and over for an hour or so during the performance of some menial household task or other.

REALiTY AND BELiEF
Reality, as you experience it, will conform to your beliefs about how it is.

If you believe your world to be dangerous and hostile, it will conform to that picture and throw up ample proof of danger and hostility to justify your position. If you believe your world to be peaceful and munificent, it will conform to that picture and produce enough abundance and harmony to prove you right. On a personal level, someone's behaviour towards you will conform to your beliefs about how that person 'is'.

In plain terms, see someone as an asshole and that's how they'll act towards you. Yet, look to the core and see the angel in them, and that's who they'll be (obviously this art requires consistent practice). Unconsciously we all mirror each other's beliefs.

Project your negative beliefs on to a situation or person and you get a negative experience. Project positive and you get positive (so get positive!).

And you can go one better. Contain your energy, suspend your judgement and project nothing, from a space of compassion, with no thought to the result, and you get miracles.

Miracles are quantum phenomena, processes of manifestation growing exponentially of themselves, meaning they get stronger as they gather steam. The opposite of a miracle is a mess. Messes are a toxic build-up of negative thought projections on a mass scale.

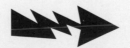

BELiEF
You are under no obligation to continue in beliefs you've grown out of.

Imagine if you could meet reality with no beliefs, just like a baby. You would simply experience things. Things would no longer be good or bad, perhaps pleasurable or painful but then, without beliefs about pleasure and pain, this wouldn't matter to you much. You might notice, perhaps, how many inappropriate beliefs you'd adopted from others and how your mind had a preset, formed opinion according to this belief system, for every experience you'd encounter.

These opinions of yours seriously limit your experience and range of available responses.

Reality can only deliver its unexpected magic when you give it room to do so. This requires you be willing to look at least partly through eyes unclouded by preconceptions. Have the humility and good grace to acknowledge that though you may have learned a fair bit while spinning round the sun, you're not omniscient, some of your beliefs may be inappropriate, and that you could be well advised to suspend them for the duration of this book, at least.

In Zen, (the Japanese art of living in the moment), they call this state of suspended belief 'beginner's mind'. Without it your experience will inevitably be preconditioned, limited and partially stale. With 'beginner's mind' you experience the news as it's happening to you faster than you ever could on CNN.

This is not to suggest you revert to the helpless newborn state and relinquish all discriminative powers but rather that you simply be willing to accept that reality, as you perceive it, is merely an opinion and not a fact.

You cannot experience reality as an objective fact because, for one thing your very presence here changes it. And that is as it's meant to be. In this experiment you are not a separate observer looking in from the outside, but an inseparable part of the whole looking out from the inside.

Reality can only be experienced subjectively and not objectively because, in practice, it's impossible to rid yourself of opinions for long enough. That is unless you're a mountain-bound yogic master and you've learned to return your mind permanently to the state of undifferentiated absoluteness. Even then I'm not so sure you wouldn't scream aloud if someone shoved a red-hot poker up your bum.

Nevertheless, it's valid training remembering that there's far more going on here than you're consciously aware of, an entire universe worth to be precise, and that your reality-limiting, preconditioned opinions are merely that and not necessarily Divine Truth.

As an experiment, temporarily suspend your beliefs about reality. Take a chance and make a few holes in the particular life-tapestry you've woven, so the reality behind it can breathe a little. Repeat this affirmation sequence in written, sung or spoken form at least nine times a month:

My experience is merely a product of my beliefs.

I am willing to suspend my beliefs temporarily.

I now remove all limitations I've placed on reality.

I am now willing to see everything with fresh eyes.

I allow my reality continuously to regenerate itself.

Note any cynical backlash from your mind and repeat the affirmation sequence once more.

Reality becomes truly exciting when you notice that it's not just you playing this game.

FOCUS
What you focus on grows.

Focus on what's positive about your life and the miracle expands, focus on the negative and the mess expands.

When you weigh up your creative, life-enhancing qualities with your destructive, life-negating tendencies, whichever aspect you pay most attention to will dominate you.

This also applies to your picture of the world at large. It's easy to find justification for holding up your view of the world in a negative light. However, with a deft little mental manoeuvre, you can just as easily see the positive. You might read the Sunday papers, for example, and come away thinking the whole world is full of corruption, violence, murder and disaster. If you focus on this view it will grow and the world will reflect your view.

On the other hand, you could focus on how the majority of people lead relatively peaceful lives and how few disasters there are compared to the size of the population. When you consider, for instance, the unthinkably enormous volume of traffic on the world's roads in any one day, and also consider the huge complexity involved in the moment-to-moment decision-making of those driving the vehicles, it is miraculous how few collisions there are.

Now apply this view to the entire global infrastructure of human society in all its ramshackle complexity. Consider the temperamental and often volatile nature of us humans, combined with our actual power to destroy (everything), and you must admit that it's a miracle in the order of the original miracle of creation that we're all still here at all.

In other words, you have the choice to create a positive world that brings pleasure to you and those affected by your life (which ultimately is everyone), or a negative one that ruins everyone's day.

As an exercise in making your reality positive, try this meditation:

For a few moments, attune your mind to the idea of harmony and peaceful co-existence flowing among all people and all nations.

The source of this idea is deep within your heart.

As you calmly breathe in and out, picture it radiating from you like a fine, coloured vapour gradually covering the face of the Earth.

See it enter the hearts of everyone, especially those stuck in the mad zones.

Feel it circulate everywhere until it comes all the way round and back to you.

This is love in action.

The source of this love is the Tao.

Savour this and come back.

WORRY

Warrior, or worrier, you choose.

This game is fully interactive. You will be presented with a series of important life choices, upon which your future will appear, and I repeat appear, to depend. At the end of the game, however, whatever the choices you have made, and the consequences that have appeared to result, your destiny will be the same: the game will end. Whatever happens after that, immortal spirit bodies and imperishable cores notwithstanding, is anyone's guess and falls outside the responsibilities of the game provider.

At the start of the game, you will notice a 'worry' option with a gargoyle icon on the upper left hand corner of the screen. On the screen's opposite corner, you'll find a ' trust 'option with a leprachaun icon. These options will not affect the series of choices you have to make, and are merely to add tone to your experience of playing the game.

If you click on the gargoyle, you go through the game feeling nervous and anxious, which releases unnecessary portions of extra adrenalin, draining your reserves, weakening your immune system, leaving you susceptible to psychic, physical and viral attack, fuzzing up your immediate atmosphere with positive ions, and thus generally making you a drag for other players to be around. If you click on the leprechaun, you go through the game feeling relaxed and confident, which releases extra chi into your system, strengthening your immune system, leaving you protected from psychic, physical and viral invasion, lighting up your immediate atmosphere with radiant tranquillity and thus making you popular at work and social gatherings.

You are free to switch between these two whenever you want, but remember this only affects the feeling-tone, and hence, quality of the experience, and will not in any way affect the actual sequence of events or final score.

Many players click on the gargoyle option as little youths, usually on advice of more 'experienced' players, and often forget the leprechaun option altogether. Remember, this game is entrancing and produces a form of intoxicated, selective amnesia in the player, which sometimes makes it hard to remember the option availability.

Worrying is nothing more than a conditioned, knee-jerked, reflexive reaction on your part to the life choices which present themselves during the passage of your personal stroll along the Great Thoroughfare. Being a worrier is merely an habitual stance you adopt. You are free to exchange it for the stance of the trusty, trusting warrior any time you choose.

Putting this choice into effect, however, requires constant vigilance as the system often tends to default to 'worry' automatically. The process of attaining zero worry status takes between approximately two nano-seconds and forty-six years to complete, depending on how many times you forget.

DOUBT

Doubting is an indulgence, which however tempting, is best avoided at all times, especially in extreme emergencies.

Doubting is what you do when you question the choice or choices you made that got you into the position in which you currently find yourself. Obviously, this is a complete waste of your energic resources. The situation, pleasant or otherwise, in which you currently find yourself, or if you like, the one into which your Tao has delivered you, is, according to the immutable law of appropriateness, exactly the right one for you at the moment. Thus all choices made by your former selves that got you here, must, by extension, have been correct. In other words, trust yourself. Trust yourself at all times, whatever the mess you seem to have generated around you, and then trust yourself some more. It's the only sensible thing to do. You make your choices and consequences arise, which you turn to your advantage wherever possible, while helping others as you go.

Trust is the only antidote to doubt. This means trusting the innate wisdom of both yourself and therefore the way you're on (your own personal Tao).

Simply repeat this affirmation continuously over the next three and a quarter days or until it becomes a repetitive pattern in the wallpaper of your mind:

I trust myself, etc.

YiELDiNG AND STiCKiNG
if you don't want negative energy to impact on you, stop resisting it.

Resisting oncoming force, whether physical, verbal or psychic, will cause an explosion in your energy field at the point of impact, which will upset your overall equilibrium and reduce your ability to respond effectively. If you provide no surface for that force to impact upon, that force will exhaust itself.

Yielding to the force of an oncoming blow, whether from something physical like a fist, or from something really nasty like the telephone bill, is like a matador elegantly side-stepping a charging bull.

Sticking is like holding your cape over the bull's face as it charges past you. Yielding means to evade oncoming force while maintaining your centre and preserving your equilibrium and dignity. Sticking means covering, that is, following the opponent with your mind, enabling you to counter instantaneously as soon as the opportunity arises. (It's all done with an intricate system of pulleys and ropes.)

Yielding and sticking are an extension of empty and full [see *Full and Empty* p. 17].

Imagine you have an opponent standing directly in front of you. Your opponent punches to the right side of your chest with her (full) left fist. Keeping your feet planted, you turn your upper body, at the waist, to your right, thus emptying your right side. This yielding motion moves the right side of your chest out of range of your opponent's strike and thus empties its force. At the same time, by turning your upper body to the right, your left side has swung round to the right also, thus enabling you to counterstrike at your opponent's right side with your left fist. Thus through yielding and sticking (alternating empty and full), the oncoming attack is returned from whence it came by its own force.

All force that comes to you is initially an expression of absolute love, pure energy that has been more or less distorted by the particular set of filters of the person who sent it. Looking past the distortion and seeing absolute love coming at you, however cruelly delivered, you simply return it unopened to sender.

It's the same with psychic or verbal attack. That oncoming force whether carried in fist, word or thought, starts initially as a pure impulse from the other to reach out to you. It only becomes violent when it passes through the filters of your opponent's personality. Look past the level of personality to the pure spirit behind, whose only currency is absolute love, and give love from your spirit to theirs. Take the negative force past you and return love.

So when that phone bill arrives, maintain your centre, don't resist it. Take it as an expression of absolute love that enables you to keep talking, and return that bill with your cheque likewise.

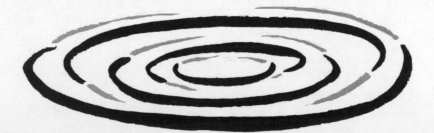

FOUR OUNCES (110 gms)
in life, three ounces of pressure is too little, five ounces is too much; four ounces, meanwhile, is just right.

When your mind and body are supple and adaptable enough that you can yield to all oncoming force, physical or otherwise, while maintaining your composure and equilibrium, thereby offering no resistance, that force will have no impact on you. The idea is never to allow oncoming force to impact on you with more or less than four ounces (110 grammes) of pressure while simultaneously standing your ground. So if a force of a thousand pounds comes at you, you yield enough to prevent that force from impacting with more than four ounces on your person. Imagine yourself standing in a pipe. A large body of water is slowly flowing down the pipe towards you. If you stand face on to it and try to resist the oncoming current, you will be knocked over as the superior force meets your resistance. If however, you turn your body sideways so that the water has less body surface to impact on, you'll be more able to hold your ground.

If someone punches your left cheek with a thousand pounds of force, but you turn it further to the left (yield), thereby emptying it immediately before full impact, you'll reduce the amount of pressure on your cheek to four ounces (but you've got to be good). It's like pulling a thousand-pound bull by exerting a light four-ounce tug on the ring through its nose.

Imagine a sparrow trying to take off from the palm of your hand but, because you're only giving it four ounces of resistance, it can't.

Conversely, when you apply pressure in any situation, apply it in measures of no more or less than four ounces. When you wallop a child's balloon with a 'thousand pounds', there's less pressure exerted over a greater surface area, causing the balloon to move only a short distance and stall. When you flick that balloon with your finger using only four ounces, you are applying more pressure pro rata over a smaller surface area, thereby enabling it to sail gracefully across the room, then stall. Same with throwing a paper airplane.

This is because focusing your intention and chi on a single point with only four ounces produces a far stronger reaction than walloping a big surface area with a thousand pounds of force.

Let your impact on others, their minds, bodies and spirits, be no more than four ounces. Ease off [see Easing Off *p. 59].*

When you speak, send the sound vibrations into the waves with no more than four ounces.

When you make physical contact (of any kind) with someone exert no more than four ounces.

When you walk or run, let your feet fall with no more than four ounces.

Four ounces allows you to listen with your whole body and thus be able to interpret the energy patterns you're listening to. Three ounces is too little and five ounces is too much for intelligent contact.

Obviously four ounces is a metaphor signifying lightness and stealth of thought, word and deed [see *Stealth* p. 98].

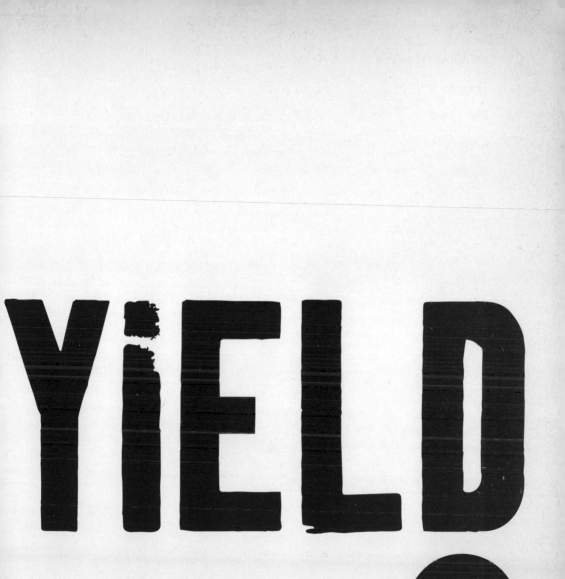

STEALTH

Always move with stealth like a watchful fox. Make your footsteps silent and let every step carry respect for the ground which supports you.

Think your footsteps light, a warrior does not clomp about like a drunken elephant. Lightening your step will not only save your shoe leather/rubber and will enable you to walk without disturbing the delicate field of sonic vibrations surrounding you, but will also help keep your energy and consequently your thoughts and emotions lighter and more level.

Next time you're walking down the street with nothing more pressing on your mind, visualise a cup of tea in your tantien (the psychic centre below your navel). Your challenge is to retain all the tea in the cup as you walk, without spilling a single drop.

Or:

Imagine the ground is covered in gold leaf and your challenge is to walk without tearing it.

With practice you'll be able to appear suddenly, as if by magic, without any sonic vibrational warning.

You enter each situation without telegraphing your arrival and leave without a trace. This ability is linked with the skill to make yourself invisible and with the ability to contain your energy.

The lightness of your step relates directly to the lightness of your energy, emotions and thoughts and vice versa, though lightness does not mean airiness. Every footstep must make intelligent contact with the ground. The soles of your feet are important receptors which collect information from the ground.

Everything that happens on this planet, from a small fly landing on your nose to a nuclear device being detonated, causes vibrations, both in the air and in the ground. These vibrations carry complex information which is assimilated automatically by your unconscious, instinctual mind. This is how animals can sense an impending earthquake – and you have this same ability.

This quality of listening through your feet is a major component of your potential psychic power. To develop it try this walking meditation:

Imagine you've gone out and bought two state-of-the-art microphones and had one installed in the sole of each foot. Yes, it would be a strange thing to do; nevertheless, as you walk along imagine these microphones are picking up the information carried in the vibrations in the ground. When your thoughts are fairly still you may receive information translated into pictures which will help guide you on your way.

This is part of the process of sensitising your body as a vibration receptor, like buying a bigger satellite dish, in order to receive a broader spectrum of information and hence increase your powers of intuition.

RUNNiNG

As a warrior, just like any other animal, you have to be able to run away from danger, if only from the danger of your own madness.

Stands to reason that sometimes in the face of extreme immediate danger you have to yield, and the only way to do that is to run. In fact, whenever you have the opportunity to run from certain danger, do it. Running away is the primary form of self-defence. What may stop you doing that is fear of losing face. However, you're much more likely to lose your face if you have to fight, so it's important that your running function is exercised with enough regularity to keep the mechanism primed. Running is not only important for this primal purpose of evading oncoming force, such as that of wild animals, wild people and even wild buses, but also for that other primal purpose of hunting, as in running to catch that wild bus.

If you're blessed with the use of your legs, running is not only an essential warrior survival skill, but also provides the perfect milieu for meditation, ie, altered state practice. Running for altered states, otherwise known in Taoist circles as 'flying on land', requires you relax, sink, breathe and feel what's going on inside you as you go, rather than straining to compete, lose weight, get fit or keep up with your running mates.

Best time of day for 'flying on land' is in the morning before the day's fumes have built up and the chi coming off the ground is still fresh.

Best place for initially practising 'flying on land' is a running track, worst (or at least the most boring) is a treadmill.

Best running partner is yourself. Company of others during a run is usually distracting and often necessitates engaging in superfluous chat which messes up your breathing and spoils your meditation.

Dress with an appropriate number of layers to ward off cold, damp, wind or heat. Do not put yourself in a position of having to run faster than you'd like just to get warm.

Wear shoes which enable you to feel your feet and spread your toes, while supporting your ankles and instep, and cushioning your soles. Alternatively, go barefoot.

Be sure your body is well warmed before starting, especially in the colder months. Any exercise system that loosens your joints, stretches your muscles and gets your awareness into your body will suffice but, generally speaking, the Taoist warm up/down exercises are the best I know (subject of future book).

Determine the route and duration of your intended course, and be clear about your intention to follow through. For example, if you decide to go nine laps of the track, make that a contract and don't break it unless you have to (not just laziness).

Visualise yourself completing the run feeling cleansed, relaxed, refreshed and reborn (why not!).

Before breaking from walk into run, check your posture for unnecessary stress, especially around the shoulder girdle and back of your neck.

Lengthen your spine, broaden your shoulders and hips, sink, raise the spirit of vitality to the top of your head, centre yourself, and relax.

Maintain this state throughout the run by running a checklist every three and a quarter minutes or so.

Commence running slowly, elbows extended away from your body, shoulders dropped, and immediately begin four-stage breathing [see Four-Stage Breathing p. 27], timing each of the four-stages to coincide with a footstep, as in breathe in, pause, in, breathe out, pause, out, in time with step, step, step, step.

Pay attention to the soles of your feet [see Your Feet p. 37], and let your mind drift. Imagine the Earth is your treadmill and you're peddling the ground beneath you so the Earth moves while you stay still. Let the pressure with which your feet pound the ground be no more than four ounces.

Run slowly, never push your pace, you're not in a race. Sprinting must come of itself like a horse opening up into a canter then a gallop, and must not be forced. When this occurs naturally, let your stride lengthen and relax your body even more, especially around the hips, feel your spirit body lift you up and fly.

For the best flights, run lightly, stealthily, and joyfully so you don't rumble the ground too much.

When you feel you're in a totally effortless groove, scoop some loop [see Scoopin' The Loop p. 49] and check in on your tantien situation [see The Three Tantiens p. 41].

On coming to the end of your run, maintain four-stage breathing as you slow down to a walk, and keep it going for a while at the original tempo to help make the transition smoother.

SPONTANEiTY
Spontaneous action is irresistible.

Spontaneous action occurs when you follow the urges that prompt you from deep within your lower tantien. Spontaneous action occurs through free will. It begins with a build-up of chi in your lower tantien (ocean of energy in your lower abdomen) which makes you feel restless if you try to ignore it. This restlessness generates a charge which travels up into your middle tantien (crimson palace in your chest), and becomes an abstract feeling of desire, as in 'I want something but I don't know what it is'. This desire itself builds up a charge which rises into the upper tantien (cave of original spirit in the middle of your brain) and is transformed by your mind into a picture of the thing to be acted out, say, of star-jumping down the street loudly singing, 'you can't always get what you want', in falsetto.

This picture then produces a charge which travels back downwards, causing a creative desire to act out in the middle tantien. This in turn generates a charge of energy in the lower tantien that finally makes you spontaneously run outside and do star-jumping with vocal accompaniment (if that's what you really want to do).

This all happens so fast you don't even notice unless you're being especially mindful. For you, it will appear as if one minute you're sitting reading a Handbook, the next you're spontaneously being a total prat out in the street.

Most urges, however, are not strong enough to go all the way up. If that initial urge in the lower tantien is only strong enough to rise to the middle tantien in your chest, you'll feel restless, wanting something you can't quite define. Your upper tantien (in your brain), being thus removed from the upthrust of energy in the lower centres, will default to an 'old, preset pictures' programme and present your mind with a series of possible actions that could satisfy that restless desire down below. As these presets are limited to past experience ie memories, they usually fall short of providing an adequate response to the urge, and you end up sitting there while some other nutter goes star-jumping and singing nonsense down the street [see *Idling vs Procrastination* p. 79].

If the middle tantien (chest) is 'blocked' through physical, emotional or psychic stress, the charge produced in the lower tantien may shoot straight into the upper tantien, bypassing the middle one, and overriding its function altogether. At this point, the original restless urge blends with a preset picture in the brain, unsupported by any true desire of the heart, which results in acting out a substitute for what should be a creative, spontaneous action, such as smoking another reefer, having another drink, seducing another lover or eating another muesli bar.

Often the urge for spontaneous action is strong but the machinery to process it isn't fully functioning because of constrictions in your tantien system. Constriction in the lower tantien, caused by stress, will distort the urge as it arises, leading to sexual blocking or excessive sexual acting out, constipation or diarrhoea, perversions and violent outbursts or extreme timidity attacks. Constriction in the middle tantien will distort the desire to act out, leading to confusion about what you want, inability to decide, coldheartedness, feeling isolated and making weird choices.

Constriction in the upper tantien distorts the pictures your mind throws up, leading to acting out things that end you up in prisons or psychiatric units. Spontaneous actions are actions of virtue [see *Virtue* p. 197] resulting from the unified totality of yourself, ie, you in full warrior mode, and can only truly arise from strong inner structure such as you can develop by practising the methods in this Handbook.

To experiment with developing spontaneity, observe how and where (not why) you block spontaneity without attempting to change that and repeat this affirmation in written and spoken form many times over the next two days:

'I am allowing spontaneous action to emerge from deep within my belly. It's safe to follow the spontaneous promptings of my body.'

Look, sod all that, being spontaneous means when you really want to do something . . . do it, and don't blame me for the consequences!

CONTAINING THE OPPOSITES
You no longer have to choose between being a villain and a saint. Now you can be both at the same time.

You don't have to choose between being confused or clear, mad or sane, loving and cold, or open-minded and rigid. As with all things yin and yang, these terms are relative, not absolute. You can be a yoga teacher who smokes, a prostitute who studies meditation and spiritual treatises, or a drug dealer who saves people's lives. You can even be an honest politician, but it's unlikely.

In this new pick 'n' mix reality, you're entirely free to admit to yourself that you contain all kinds of pairs of opposites. According to the immutable law of yin and yang, every human quality has its opposite number lurking on the dark side of its moon. According to the world of fairy tales upon which the paradigm of our dying culture is based, a person, and especially a warrior person, is either noble or ignoble. But if he's only noble, what about the time he didn't quite tell the truth to his girlfriend, and if he's ignoble, what about all the people he's helped? It's impossible to be simply one or the other. Come out! Acknowledge that you're containing all the opposites, contradictions and paradoxes of the world within you.

Same with another person. Don't judge them as being this or that because, depending on lighting and camera angle, it is quite clear that they are this-that. Same with situations. A particular situation cannot be good or bad. It depends entirely on where and when you're looking from, and who's looking. A situation is both good and bad. Even the silver linings of clouds can be extremely tarnished.

Acceptance of this leads you to stop jumping to conclusions and to observe yourself, other people and the situations that develop between you, without judgement. Once you can see that you, another person, or a situation is neither good nor bad but both, your perspective is instantaneously raised to the transpersonal level which transcends opposites. When you transcend the opposites, you are dealing directly with the Tao, and are for that time worthy of being called master or mistress.

List all your positive qualities, then list their opposites.

List all your negative qualities, then list their opposites.

List the two groups of opposites and see if they tally.

Say, 'I contain all these contradictions. I am this and that. I can be a hero and a coward, a healer and a dealer, an angel and a demon, happy and sad, confident and terrified, love myself and hate myself, all at the same time, and still be perfectly sane.'

Now stop all this shit and go out and do something interesting.

Although you're free to admit these contradictions to yourself, you may not always be free to do so in public. Sometimes the game demands you make a show of tying your colours to the flagpole. At these times, while fully honouring the game, remind yourself of the relativity of all phenomena and don't believe your own opinions, as this will limit the possibilities inherent in the situation.

MORALiTY VS AMORALiTY
Morals make the moron.

Traditionally, the way of morality, of observing the mores, was the Confucianist path. The followers of old Kung Fu Tse (Confucius), meaning 'kung fu master', believe that if you teach a person a set of behavioural responses to match every possible situation, their inner psycho-emotional structure will adapt itself to conform to that outer shape. In other words, shape the external and the internal will conform.

There is obviously some validity to this scheme. Vast totalitarian empires have indeed flourished for a while on this same principle. It requires a large and comprehensive set of rules and precepts to be learned and strictly obeyed. To enforce this, the individual is obliged to police both themselves and others, thereby creating the grass roots of a police state. These rules or morals, if strictly adhered to, are intended to mould your character into one of virtue. This does not allow for the fact that every person contains all possible contradictions and thus relies on suppression and denial of the shadow side to be in any way effective.

To uphold a system like this, which depends on force to maintain appearances, is like trying to build your house from scratch by starting with painting the walls. Just as vast totalitarian states which rely on inordinate portions of force to maintain order eventually crumble and fall, so too do individuals who, by concentrating exclusively on externals at the expense of their inner integrity, end up having nervous breakdowns, starting wars, abusing whores and causing all manner of unnecessary mischief. It is no accident that the words 'moral' and 'morose' share the same etymological root in that by blindly following the mores you lose touch with your true nature and become morose. Hence morals make the moron.

The wayward followers of Tao, by contrast, believe that to modify your behaviour you must attend to the development of your true nature by focusing your attention inwards. In time, through diligent practice of inner principles and methods presented in this very Handbook, you will attain a state of perpetual peace, absolute inner harmony, limitless power and eternal duration [see *The Three Friendly Deities Visualisation* p. 44]. When in this state, even if only for a temporary stop-over, you are moving with your true nature, which is intrinsically life-affirming and positive. When you move with your true nature, which comprises the very essence of your spirit body, you are automatically in a state of virtue, ie, authenticity. When you are authentic, all your thoughts and actions towards self and others will be true, and hence life-enhancing.

Morals then become unnecessary and irrelevant. When you are moving with your true nature, your three tantiens are working together in unison and three-part harmony, your heart is open, your mind is clear and your actions spontaneous, you cannot fail to treat yourself and other people with absolute care and respect to the best of your ability at the time. Additionally, understanding the significance of the law of cause and effect, ie, act unto others as you would have them act unto you, provides a secondary check on any unbridled action of yours.

As a warrior you need no morals, rules or precepts, other than to respect kindly all life as much as your own; to respect kindly your own life as if it is the universe itself; to help and heal yourself and others whenever you can; and to inflict minimum damage in love affairs and acts of genuine self defence against those threatening to damage or destroy your person or dependants.

PRESENT MOMENT AWARENESS
There is only one moment and that's the one happening now, as you sit here reading this.

This has always been the only moment and always will be. This moment never changes. What changes is the scenery occurring around this moment. This moment has seen the birth and demise of a hundred universes and will probably hang around to watch the birth and demise of a few hundred more. But whatever the time on your clock or date on your calendar, this moment will never change.

Rein in the wild horses of your mind as they charge unbridled hither and thither, into remembered scenes of the past or imagined scenes of the future. Draw your awareness backwards into the cave of your original spirit, and centre yourself in this moment, now.

Resist the temptation to project your mind willy nilly into an imagined future except during positive visualisation sessions [see *Visualisation* p. 122]. Projecting even five minutes into the future often leads to anxiety if your thoughts are left to roam freely. For example, you're looking forward to your friend coming round. You project an imaginary scene on to your inner screen. You see the tea and cakes, the ambience, the chit chat, the love shared, and you feel happy as your chi rises to your middle tantien (heart centre). There you are, milking the fantasy, when all of a sardine, your system defaults to the 'worry' option [see *Worry* p. 90]. At this juncture the worry gargoyle infiltrates the happy tone of your moment, you start getting anxious, and your fantasy turns to horror as you picture your friend arriving in uncommunicative mood, the tea being cold, the cakes stale, the ambience flat, the chit chat strained and the love refused.

Meantime, while you've been playing with your adrenalin levels, this moment has been continuing in its majestic way as the scenery shifts all around it, and you've missed it all. This moment is all there is, and you've missed it.

It's the same with memories of the past. When you let your mind dive into past pictures for too long, whether to nourish yourself on nostalgia or punish yourself with regrets, you inevitably eventually end up with an unsettling feeling of unfulfilled longing. Meanwhile, the scenery's passing you by and you've lost precious time not being here.

The fact is that all the power in the universe that ever was and ever will be is contained in this present moment. This power (chi) is the catalyst that transforms your thoughts into manifest reality. When your mind is focused in another time, you're denied access to this power, and therefore deprived of the very nourishment you're erroneously seeking in past and future projections.

Other than for dedicated visualisation sessions to heal past or future scenarios, spending time anywhere other than this present moment constitutes insanity. Only in the stillness of this moment can you find the power to manifest the things you want. Only in this present moment will you find the nourishment, peace and healing you're craving.

This eternal moment is like a pool containing the waters of youth and immortality. When your mind is not occupied with thoughts (memories and future projections, regrets and worries) and you're breathing freely in a centred, meditative state, it's like bathing in these healing waters.

You can only be truly sane in this moment. In fact, you can only be truly anything in this moment.

SELF-PiTY

Unless you or yours are currently facing a firing squad or such-like (in which case, why are you reading this now?), the only thing blocking you from your perfect happiness and fulfilment in this present moment is self-pity.

Self-pity is a device you use unconsciously to prevent yourself fully engaging in the present moment and moving on in your life. It is a delay tactic, originating from fear of the new, and hence lack of trust in the wisdom of your particular journey down the Great Thoroughfare.

Danger with self-pity is, it drains your chi, robs you of your spirit and it's insidious. It's a virus in the system which creeps in unnoticed through the cracks in your psychic structure like a poisonous vapour and fills the mental space in your upper tantien. It gets everywhere, and just like the fourteen pounds per square inch pressure of air around you now, you don't notice it unless you're being particularly vigilant. Being parasitical by nature, it attaches itself to whichever host-thought is running past your screen at the time. Being in this way invisible, only taking on the visible form of its host-thought, it is a master shapeshifter, and thus nearly impossible to detect. Though it comes in many guises, it often dresses up as the sensible voice of reason, having a go at the injustices of your life. It will throw ideas up like, 'This is completely ridiculous and shouldn't be happening' [see *Trust* p. 84], or, 'I'm tired, I can't be assed' [see *Idling vs Procrastination* p. 79], or 'What's the point, the world's going to end anyway' [see *End-of-the-World-Phobia* p. 119]. Being disguised thus as the sensible voice of mature reason, it is entirely plausible, and will get you every time, until you learn to recognise it.

The only tell-tale sign is that you feel unhappy. It's that simple.

You may think unhappiness is inevitable or somehow obligatory, but even in times of extreme distress, grief, fear, sorrow, for example, you can still choose to be perfectly happy and fulfilled in your core while you experience the pain of the moment [see *Containing the Opposites* p. 104].

Your best friend may have just died and your whole body is racked with the most profound sobs of abject grief; you can, if you so choose, simultaneously feel an imperishable core of happiness in your centre [see *Centring* p. 30] as you recognise the perfect harmony of the Tao. Choosing otherwise in this or any other such distressing situation, in other words losing your positive attitude, is an act of self-pity.

Maintaining a positive attitude, and remaining centred in this present moment at all times, and at all costs, is the antidote.

The real beauty of this particular game, however, is that once you've recognised self-pity, it vanishes (till the next time) and you get such a blast of creative positivity by contrast that you can't help jumping up with a hop, skip and a whistle, and doing something new.

IWT (the Institute of Wayward Taoism) recommends conducting twenty-three minutes' duration self-pity sessions whenever you're feeling particularly unhappy. Designate the allotted time as being for self-pitying thoughts and feelings only. Under no circumstances allow in a single positive thought or feeling for the duration of the session. Allow yourself to wallow fully in self-pity's murky waters. Rub it in your hair and in your eyes. As soon as the twenty-three minutes is up, however, stop. Stop indulging and be happy.

DISPELLING NEGATIVITY
When you overcome your preferences, the Tao in all its liberating majesty, can sometimes be glimpsed in a turd more easily than in a breathtaking sunset.

What follows is the 'I love doggy-do on my shoe' meditation. Beset by a self-pity attack of the 'I hate this' variety, as in, 'I hate this day, I hate this feeling of dejection, I hate this dog turd on my shoe, I hate feeling lonely and scared like this', you admit that in your secret heart of hearts, beneath the layers of mental conditioning, you're actually loving every phenomenon that pokes its head in your face, because it's happening in your life. You love the whole messy, smelly, dark, dingy, rank, mildewed, viral, rancid euuchh about it because, beneath your surface layer of conditioned (Pavlovian) reflexes, as in 'I'm not supposed to like dog shit on my shoe - I'm not supposed to enjoy the smell', you secretly find the shock of the slide, 'oh, shit', the mild embarrassment, the fear of being ostracised, and the tartness of the smell, quite exhilarating.

This is what happens when you surrender to the Tao, by investing in the loss of that particular layer of conditioned reflexes (it makes you weird!). Obviously it doesn't do to get carried away with this investment and go sliding around in dog shit all day, as this would offend others who might not be at such an advanced stage of practice as you.

So next time that dread thing happens to you, simply perform the 'I love doggy-do's on my shoes' meditation, and you may shock yourself with the extent to which you can let go of prejudices and ultimately liberate yourself from the self-limiting realm of preferences.

To practise it now, simply go about your daily doings as usual. During the course of your day/night, you will see, hear, smell, taste, touch and think about many phenomena you'd normally reject automatically. Instead, catch yourself each time, and say, 'I love this', as in, 'I love this day, I love this feeling of dejection, I love this doggy-do on my shoe (in theory!), I love this noise of drilling outside my window, I love those car fumes, I love having to write this and not being able to go out and play in the sunshine.'

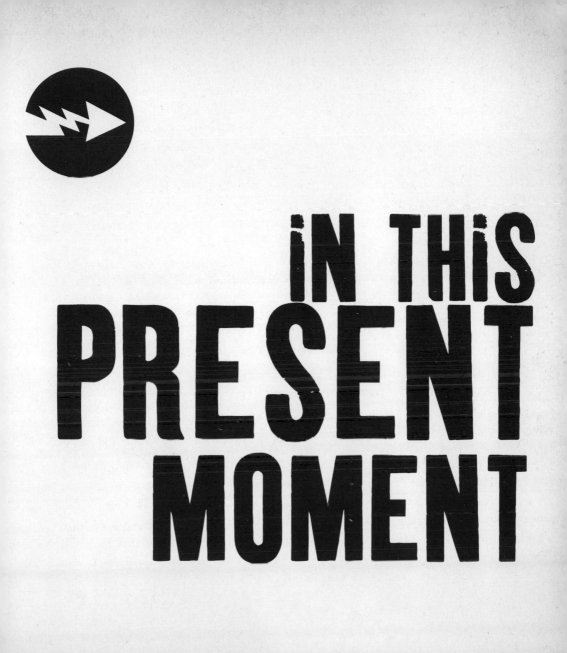

At first, you just pretend but if you're really mindful and honest you may, in time, notice how your heart can open to absolutely anything if you strip away that layer of conditioned reflexes which prevents your spontaneous enjoyment of everything in your life.

Of course, when you voluntarily enter a state of suspended judgement like this, you are still free to use your powers of discrimination, ie, avoid that slide for a smell-free ride.

VULNERABiLiTY
Feeling vulnerable does not diminish your abilities or effectiveness as a warrior. in fact, it increases them.

A phase of heightened vulnerability usually occurs when you're forced to let go of someone or something that you were using to help shore you up a little. This exposes the deficiency you were compensating for by using that person or thing to prop you up. When you've been leaning on a rotten wall (lover, job, bad habit, etc), and the wall suddenly collapses, you are momentarily unbalanced and it is in this period, while striving to retrieve your balance, that you feel unsupported and vulnerable.

Vulnerability, however, is the only authentic state. Being vulnerable means being open, for wounding but also for pleasure. Being open to the wounds of life means also being open to the bounty and beauty. Don't mask or deny your vulnerability, it is your greatest asset. Be vulnerable, quake and shake in your boots with it. The new goodness that is coming to you, in the form of people, situations and things, can only come to you when you're vulnerable, ie, open.

Picture yourself as a vulnerable little youth, sitting in the middle of a huge protective cosmic egg. Although you are gently trembling as you prepare to make your transition into a new phase, you have the courage to be open and vulnerable. See yourself drop your heavy adult armour and surrender to the unknown.

STABILISING – STANDING CONTEMPLATION
Stand up like a tree and be counted!

Before you can think straight you have to stabilise yourself. Otherwise it's like trying to use your powerbook/lap-top with someone rocking and rolling it around in front of your eyes. Before you can go into the 'clear thinking' program you've got to steady that box o' ones and noughts just to be able to see the icon to click on.

To stabilise your system just so you can think clearly, take yourself outside, having ensured adequate and appropriate layers of protective clothing have been draped about and fitted to your person, and find a spot where you can trance out in relative seclusion.

Stand with your feet at about the width of your shoulders, perhaps a little wider, with the outsides of your feet parallel, both feet facing directly forwards. Bend your knees a little (one over each foot), making sure they don't bow inwards, and tilt your sacrum forwards a bit so it feels like you're sitting on a bar-stool. Check your posture, suspend your head [see Raising the Spirit of Vitality p. 39], *sink and relax. Keeping your shoulders down, slowly raise your arms to the level of your chest and shape them like you're holding a huge tree-trunk you can't quite get your hands to meet around. Turn your palms inwards to face you, and maintain a space of about one grapefruit between them.*

Extend through your shoulders, elbows, wrists and fingertips, curving your arms so you can reach round the tree.

Keep checking your relaxation factor level in key locations: back of neck, face, chest and belly. Imagine chi dripping off the underside of your arms, like thick golden fluid. Feel everything very heavy and tending to sink downwards, while your spine lengthens upwards through the top of your head to the heavens, holding you upright. Keep checking the bend and openness of your knees and keep your shoulders down, ie not unnaturally raised.

Lock your skeletal structure into position and allow your bones to support you in the shape.

Hold this shape for the length of nine phases of four-stage breathing the first day, then eighteen the next and so on until you can stand for eighty-one rounds.

At this stage, introduce scoopin' the loop, and three tantien visualisation [see Scoopin' the Loop *p. 49 and* Three Tantiens *p. 41].*

Approach this gently and not as a he/she-man challenge. Do not try to suppress the subtle internal movements that want to occur of themselves inside your body. Involuntary shaking, if it should occur, signifies a healthy release of tension and should be fostered, encouraged and enjoyed.

If you stand every day for at least eighty-one breath cycles (some spiritual maniacs stand for an hour or more), you will strengthen your physical and energetic base and develop rapid stabilising ability (RSA), which will enable you to retrieve your stability more quickly in a crisis. (Remember that the only difference with a master when dealing with disaster, is a master gets off it faster.)

While standing in this posture imagine that rather than a tree you're holding, it's a column of supernatural, special effects light, which is rushing downwards from the heavens, through the ring formed by your arms, deep into the centre of the Earth. As you stand channelling this force, you are receiving a mega-charge of cosmic chi.

Use this any time your thoughts are in a flurry, to settle yourself. Thank you.

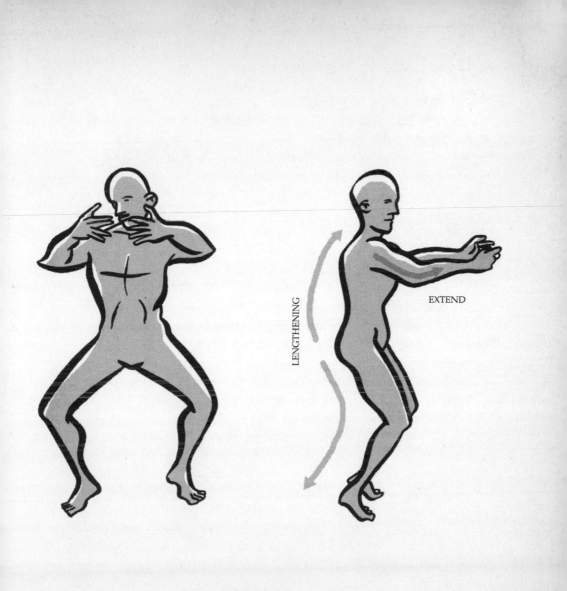

LENGTHENING

EXTEND

STABILISING

ACCLAiM

it's wonderful being acclaimed and horrible when they topple you – but only as much as you take your fictional self seriously.

Fame and ignomy merely consist of others' projections, fantasies and opinions, which mean about as much as yours. People's opinions of you are like clouds passing in the sky, pushed here and there by whichever wind is prevailing. When they're with you, your mythical self gets a massage, when they're against you, it gets punched around, but it only hurts as much as you believe in the myth of who you are.

Conversely, fame, acclaim, renown or just straightforward approval can cause tension when you're afraid to lose them, and ignomy and disgrace can be quite enjoyable as a refuge for a while.

Ultimately, it's you who does the approving and disapproving of yourself and your 'public' simply reflects that in this nutty hall of mirrors.

Approval and disapproval alternate on the revolving yin-yang wheel, so any effort to hold on to the former and avoid the latter is futile. It's far better to identify with your spirit which is eternal, unchanging and beyond anyone's approval or disapproval, even yours.

Picture yourself as a total social failure and disgrace and say to this fictitious person, 'I love you.'

Now see yourself as a very important social celebrity and say to that fictitious person, 'I love you.'

Then continue to say 'I love you' to yourself as often as you remember till you die.

At the party everyone wants to talk to you and tell you you're great, because that's their agenda. The tabloids tear you apart and that's just their agenda. If you can have the presence of mind, you don't take it personally.

Fame and infamy, approval and disapproval are illusions. Sometimes they please you, sometimes they tease you.

END-OF-THE-WORLD PHOBiA
Concerning yourself about this world coming to an end and other such catastrophes is just another way to distract yourself from the present moment.

Nobody knows when the world will end. It may end tomorrow, next week or never. Everything is in a state of flux. This is nothing new, it has always been so. Just because the world, or specifically this planet is currently dominated by humans, there is nothing to say it won't soon be dominated by spiders. For you and me this would be uncomfortable and would definitely screw up our marketing plans. For the spiders, however, it would be business as usual.

In fact, with every word you read, a world is coming to an end, as someone somewhere hangs up their Earth-boots for good, which is exactly why it's silly to waste even a moment worrying about anything, especially the end of the world, even if it does make for great romantic tragedy.

End-of-the-world phobia is a form of self-pity and is, as such, a procrastination device [see *Idling vs Procrastination* p. 79], used as a way to avoid engagement with the world that's happening around you in the present moment.

Instead of worrying and lamenting, rejoice. Rejoice in supreme gratitude for the magnificent thrill of every moment, however strenuous or weird that moment might be.

This does not mean you walk around in ignorance of the dangers facing you on this planet at this present time but simply that you don't let that prevent you from being fully alert and able to respond effectively, appropriately and cheerfully to whatever's happening in the present moment at this time. At times, fear of the danger, sadness at the needless destruction and despair at the suffering, will inevitably overwhelm you. At these times, apply yourself with redoubled vigour to doing everything you can to preserve and nurture life, and as you do that, rejoice, ie, literally feel joy again. It's the only thing for a warrior to do.

PANiC
'You must never panic, my dear.'

So you eventually decide to visit the great spiritual teacher everyone's been going on about. The deal is, after meditating at her feet for half an hour, in the company of a most earnest posse of spiritual seekers (why don't they get a life etc), you have the opportunity to ask her one question. Obviously it's got to be good: deep, meaningful and showing that you've gone through your metaphysical paces and evolved a touch beyond the 'norm'. So as soon as the opportunity presents itself, you grab it and looking innocently into her incredibly clear eyes (she's not been smoking reefers without inhaling) and with a practised tone of spontaneity, recite the question you've been rehearsing in your head all during the meditation, a question that would show you'd grappled with the notion of your own demise and had devised some even greater fear with which to torment yourself. You ask, 'At the exact moment of your death, if you panic, will that adversely affect your state of your consciousness, effectively scattering you and therefore preventing your transfer to higher planes?' A great silence fills the room. You can smell the impact on said earnest posse as the heavy import of your words begins to translate graphically. She slowly turns her head to look at you, and after a great and expectant pause, fixes you with a most sincerely penetrating stare and replies,

'You must never panic, my dear'.

Panic, as in pandemonium, is simply letting your mind run away with you. Instead of reining in the wild stallion of your mind [see *Centring* p. 30], you've allowed the bastard to break into a gallop and he's about to charge over the cliff's edge, when, if you've been reading the Handbook and paying attention, you suddenly remember to breathe [see *Breathing* p. 22]. Slowing down the tempo and allowing the movement to deepen, you snap back into your imperishable core and you're in warrior mode again. Panic over.

ORiENTATiON
As a warrior you must always know where you are.

And currently where you are is on a huge globe with a relatively thin crust of stone, containing fire in its bowels, rotating on its own slightly tilted axis, at 1,000 miles per hour, in an easterly direction while simultaneously travelling in orbit around an enormous ball of burning hydrogen, 93,000,000 miles away, at 66,000 miles per hour. That's sixty-six thousand miles per hour, or nineteen miles per second, which is much faster than you've maybe ever imagined, and means that you will be travelling nearly 60,000,000 miles this coming year.

Beauty is, you don't have to imagine it, you can feel it instead. And if you want to know what it's like, simply stop. Be still, and in that stillness, whatever you're feeling in your belly: that's it. Easy as that. This is what it feels like to go 66,000 miles per hour, while spinning at one thousand. Seems it should make you feel dizzy, but thanks to the spin, you're probably managing to maintain your equilibrium most of the time. However, at those times when you feel out of sorts and disorientated, like you're adrift all alone, without reference points, in a sea of meaningless human nonsense, one totally effective way to pop yourself back into the centre of the frame, is to pass a few moments actively contemplating the absurd speed at which you're actually hurtling, at this precise moment, through this vast vaulted arch of celestial expanse we so casually refer to as 'space'.

At those times, when this contemplation suits your mood, a mere seven minutes' worth will suffice to clear your perspective and bring your mind back to the wonder of what's actually going on around here, beneath the distractions of daily human doings. It will also hopefully inspire awe and maybe dread, which is useful in reminding you to appreciate the great benefits of having somewhere relatively solid to rest your sitting-bones.

See yourself at a theme park on a planet simulator, which gives you the full sensation of travelling round a sun at nineteen miles per second, while counter-spinning on its own axis at 1,000 miles per hour. The sensation is surprisingly subtle yet completely sublime. You remain transfixed for the entire duration of the ride, which lasts a full seven minutes. You then get off the simulator, leave the theme park, and carry on with the things you like to do.

Invest some time and energy in practising this orientation contemplation, until you can do it in the on-the-spot, flash-on, flash-off, tune-in-at-a-moment's-notice style, in the course of a busy day's crossing from sunrise to sunset.

ViSUALiSATiON
You have to see something clearly before you can manifest it.

Visualisation is the ritual of focusing your concentration on an image of something you want and seeing it as if it's already manifested.

This image can be graphic, symbolic or a combination of both. You may want peace of mind, for example, in which case you can focus either on a graphic image of yourself, your face, your body looking peaceful, or on a symbolic image you make up, such as a sunflower sticking out of a yin-yang sign, inside a star, surrounded by pink mist, perhaps (but I do hope not – so new-age gauche!). You may want to combine these two by seeing yourself looking chilled, while you dance pirouettes on the petals of the sunflower. You may simply wish to picture the word 'peace' in 3D, prehistoric rock. The image you choose may consist of a still frame or a series of moving frames.

Sit back in your cave of original spirit in the centre of your brain like you're in a projection room, and project your image on to an imaginary screen on the inside of your forehead. Simultaneously stay connected to your imperishable core and breathe.

As you watch the projected image or series of images upon your inner screen, you invest that image with a portion of passion from your heart and chi from your belly, which is to say you focus your intention on that image until you can feel it as a reality.

Once you've felt the sensation of your image being a real life event, smelled it, tasted it, heard it and touched it, let the image shrink to the size of an atom surrounded in subtle light, say something amen-like, like 'so be it' and let it go. Letting it go means entrusting its manifestation to the Tao and easing off.

There will then be a time lag of anything from three days to thirty years depending on the viability of the scheme, strength of belief and other variables beyond my power to comprehend but which normally fall under the jurisdiction of destiny, before your image finally takes shape on the Earth plane. Visualising for acquiring or developing personal qualities such as confidence, slimness of hip, beauty of visage or warmness of heart, as well as for talents or specific skills such as mastering a new scale on the guitar or giving a rousing speech, tends to produce swifter results than visualising for acquiring £23 million, but there are absolutely no fixed rules.

Visualisation can be used with equal effectiveness for the most banal purposes like getting a parking space (buy a bicycle), or a taxi (for when it's really pissing down), and for the most profound, such as creating your own immortal spirit body [see *Spirit Body* p. 57]. It can be used for things like successful completions of projects, sales of houses, upping the circulation of a magazine, winning a race, for example, as well as for 'altruistic' concepts, like creating peaceful worlds.

If two or more people visualise the same thing simultaneously, the energy for that thing to manifest will be exponentially multiplied. That's how elections are won, ie, marketed, and religions sustained, ie, marketed.

There's not much difference between visualising and day-dreaming. Both involve bringing an image to a place inside you where you can experience it as real.

Visualisation differs from day-dreaming only in how you set it up. Whereas day-dreaming is an undisciplined ramble through the meadows of your imagination – your nation of images – visualisation is a focused foray.

BLUE LASSO
if you're wanting something new, simply chuck your blue lasso.

Imagine you wanted a fancy new top o' the range lap-top and you were setting up a visualisation to draw it into manifestation in your life. So you go through your ritual, centring, breathing, sinking, relaxing, focusing your concentration on an image of the lap-top, and what have you. Then if you want to give the ritual a sharp boost, thereby increasing its effectiveness tenfold, try this little 'blue lasso visualisation boost' tool.

When you have the image of the lap-top clearly in focus and unwavering in centre frame, picture a lasso of flashlight-blue light darting out from your lower tantien (just below your navel) and extending towards the image of the lap-top. Now surround that lap-top with it and reel it in just like a real cowboy or fisherman (depending on which metaphor you're going with).

It won't do at all to attempt this with images of other people, as when say you try to lasso a specific lover. This constitutes 'black' or manipulative magic, which must be avoided by warriors at all costs. Manipulative magic always backfires and ends up trapping you and setting you back ten lifetimes.

MANIFESTATION
THE IMPORTANCE OF OTHER PEOPLE
Everybody wants to get what they want.

Even saints want to get what they want, which is to do saintly business. There's nothing to be ashamed of in this respect. The game of getting what you want is the best distraction from the coldness of endless space we've come up with yet. It gives you a sense of purpose, which keeps you off the streets, and a sense of direction, without which you don't get out of bed. And if you don't get out of bed, you eventually shrivel and die. So getting out of bed to get what you want is good. However, if what you want, when you get it, is more harmful in the balance than healing, to yourself and others, then it's probably better to stay in bed, until you've got your heart in the right place.

Things of the world you want invariably involve other people. If it's money you're after, and there's nothing wrong with that [see *Money* p. 194], it will come to you through other people. If it's carnal or romantic love you want, unless you're odd, it will come through other people. If it's a vast creative project you're wishing to bring to fruition, it will occur through other people.

The obvious way then to get what you want is to somehow persuade other people to give it to you. This is usually done through a variety of means, both

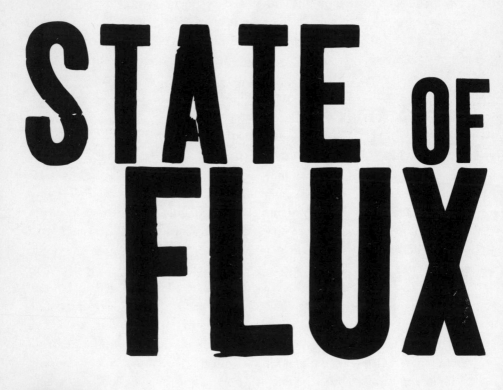

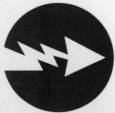

overt and covert, including begging, pleading, advertising, the threat or use of brute force and just plain shmoozing. These are all external methods, requiring specialised skills and consistent application, and which rely on brute force, as opposed to the internal, which merely require an ability to focus, and rely on chi.

It so happens that the IWT (Institute of Wayward Taoism) conducted extensive experiments which concluded overwhelmingly that the internal approach to getting what you want was a pretty convincing twenty-three per cent more energy efficient and cost-effective than the external approach.

The internal approach is similar to the external, in that you still get what you want through other people. Where it differs is in the level of communication you're operating on.

Things you want start off as ideas in your mind, creations of consciousness. The picture then takes form on your inner projection screen, and with a little passion from your heart and chi from your belly, becomes a thought form, which travels right to the heart of the secret machinery in the universal engine room, and in time is materialised on the Earth plane.

On the way to its full materialisation, however, this thought form has to also pass through the resistance of the minds of various other key people, who have to ratify it with their agreement.

If the energy coming off the engine room about this idea is strong enough, this agreement will come easily. If not, the idea will get snagged at the planning stage. To get the energy strong enough to go through all resistance, you have to send it out strongly enough in the first place. So that rather than put your energy into persuading others to agree with your idea (external approach), you put your energy into sending the original picture into the heart of the universal machinery.

This is a long-winded way of saying 'as you see it, so it will be', and that if when you see it, you really concentrate with passion on the picture, then send it out to the Tao, it will manifest easily and effortlessly, and save you a lot of trainer rubber.

GOiNG FOR ESSENCE
Surprise yourself.

Rather than going for the specific form of what you think you want, sometimes do the groovy Taoist thing and go for essence instead. By which I mean, rather than visualising a specific lover coming to you (manipulative – we don't talk to you!), visualise yourself with the feeling of fulfilment you think you'd get from being with that lover. Rather than visualising £23 million coming to you (visualise it coming to me!), visualise yourself with the feeling of security and satisfaction you'd have every time you received your bank statement. It's not the thing itself which you long for, it's the feeling or essence that comes with it. It's not the lover, it's the love. It's not the money, it's the security or excitement. It's not the fame, it's the feeling good enough.

When you focus on attaining the feeling you want, you create the vibration that will draw to you the kind of people, events and things that will generate, through the immutable law of affinity, that feeling in you. In this way you don't limit what the Tao can do for you by placing one of your local, personal filters on it.

Instead this is like doing a lucky dip. For some strange reason the regular programming round these parts has it that you set the day up with the proviso, 'I'll only feel OK about myself today if I achieve such and such'. The normal thing would then be to go for manifesting that such and such. If, however, you were to go for manifesting a feeling of OK-ness, whatever occurred, you'd feel OK, and such and such, or something even better, would then probably manifest on its own, and if it didn't, it wouldn't matter anyway.

Perhaps this is just a Taoist cop-out, but if you're feeling OK anyway, then what the hell.

The main advantage of this non-specific style of manifesting is that it allows for surprises which delight you, and may you have many today.

Say, 'today I am open to receiving many delightful surprises.'

EFFORTLESS ACHIEVING

Before you read this item see yourself getting to the end of it easily and effortlessly with a smile on your face. Then forget all that, relax and read the item.

You have an intention for something to occur. You visualise that eventuality with concentrated focus, imbued with a portion of passion and chi, then you let it go, like sending an e.mail. You picture what you want to say and the effect that will have on the recipient, then you write it and press send. At that point you do not try to follow it down the phone line to your local server and onwards to the server at the other end, you simply let it go and get on with the next distraction in your life.

In time your intention will go to the heart of the universal machinery and return to you in manifest form. Meanwhile you have wasted no energy on trying to make it happen, you've simply intended something and let it go. This doesn't mean you sit around like a lazy bum waiting for things to occur, unless you want to, of course. On the contrary, letting go frees you up to follow your spontaneous impulses; these are urges which appear to arise of themselves and which are too strong to ignore. Whenever you follow one, it will lead you closer to your goal (the worthiness of which depends entirely on you, so watch out!).

For example, you may be working as leader of a team of people engaged in a creative project. You wish for a particular result but the various egos involved may be pulling in different directions, causing resistance to your goal. Rather than trying to persuade and cajole your team into submission to your will, you visualise your intended result, let it go, and free yourself for spontaneous action. In the course of getting on with your work on the project, one by one, all the team members come round to your vision, meanwhile thinking of it as their own. This is known as leading from behind.

You set your intention, let it go and get on with your life and, in the fullness of time, what you intended comes to pass on its own. When this doesn't seem to work, it's either because your intention wasn't clearly focused enough, or because what you thought you wanted was in fact too limited in the greater scheme of things, and something even better's coming down the line.

JUMPING THE QUEUE
in this game you either win or you win, it's up to you.

You arrive at the club. You've arranged to meet your friends inside. To your dismay, the line of people waiting to gain access to an already packed venue stretches right around the corner.

You're not on the guest list, paying or otherwise and you're not feeling up to telling stories to the burly bouncers at the door but you have to get in.

Then you remember your newly honed skills of getting what you want by visualising it so. You centre yourself, slow down your breathing, sink your energy and stand there in the street picturing yourself walking confidently up to the bouncers. They think they recognise you as somebody or other of vaguely celebrity status and give you that special bouncer nod and you're in.

Visualisation done, you check yourself for relaxation levels and plugging in to your core energy, stride past the line of people up to the door of the club.

And it doesn't work. With not so much as a glance they turn you away like so much jetsam.

There you are in the street in a state of total embarrassment. Moreover, you feel let down by the Handbook and start to doubt the reality of your psychic power.

But the thing is, it doesn't always work, and it's important that it doesn't because it's these times that teach you the most. The process of self-examination which may ensue now is valuable.

It could just be you're wearing the wrong clothes or that your inner confidence and self-esteem is a bit low. Maybe your visualisation wasn't fully connecting with all three centres [see *The Three Tantiens* p. 41]. For sure it was in your destiny to be refused entry tonight. This would be symbolic of you delaying your own progress through the next metaphorical doorway in your life because you've more to learn first.

So you humbly join the end of the queue which is now even further away and find solace in being ordinary. From the point of view of your training, it's been a most successful night.

See the bouncer as your guru for the night, and the people in the queue as fellow devotees and say this affirmation twelve times:

'I am willing to receive the gift in every situation, however stupid I may feel.'

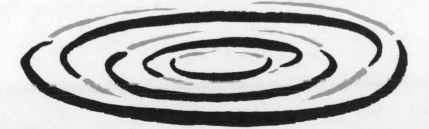

CLUB CULTURE
A packed, heaving club-full of sweaty people dancing is the perfect milieu for miracles.

So you're at the club, the music selection falls neatly into the category that suits your internal tempo tonight. Your head's done much nodding up and down. Your hips have moved with the grooves and your toes have tapped. Your eardrums have been wobbled furiously a few times by well-meaning friends and acquaintances attempting the impossible task of conducting spoken dialogue with you using the method where you take it in turns to shout down each other's ear holes. Of course you can't decipher more than a word or two which matters not as it's all crap anyway but you nod and smile and your Eustachian tubes itch.

It's around four in the morning and you're starting to wonder why you're here. The magic and whatever else you've been playing with has started to wear a little thin, holes have appeared in your trance and finally you have to admit that you're bored. Of course, you secretly imagine there must be something pathologically wrong with you because, while everyone else seems to be fully engaged in the game, you don't know what to do with yourself.

This is the perfect time to do a miracle.

Put your awareness into your heart centre, your crimson palace, the centre of transpersonal love, where that old rascal Benefactor lives. Let him radiate a steady stream of warm energy from the centre of your chest into the hearts of everyone in the club as you inhale and exhale deeply and smoothly.

Continue this for a few minutes, then stop and wait and if someone really special doesn't come up and pull you into the fun or some such pleasant occurrence, I'll put my shoes on and go home.

The point is to reframe the experience, to see through the illusion of club with clubbers having fun, to a deeper reality of spirits, come together to channel and transform some energy. Now rather than be a lost punter pretending to be happy, you're a miracle operator on a mission.

However, it is totally contraindicated to tell anyone else about what you're doing at the time or after. Not only would this be a pitiful and nauseating new age-way to grab attention but would also render the spell null and void.

AFFIRMATIONS
This is so because i say so.

Everything you manifest here starts with a thought. Thoughts have power. Words are thought containers, therefore words have power. Check it out in the media, most of what's reported in the news is about what people have said, rather than what they've done. Doing magical operations, whether in organised churches or in a meeting of the Golden Circle, depends on the correct use of words. Successful advertising depends on the correct use of words. Getting any message across from the most sublime to the most ridiculous, requires words. 'In the beginning God spoke and said let there be light' meaning that even the great dude herself had to use words before there could be vision.

Words shape worlds, which is why it's so important to use them precisely. Doing affirmations is the art of shaping your world by using precise words in a positive way. An affirmation, literally a saying 'yes' to something you want, can be spoken, sung (chanted), written or a combination of the three. An affirmation will, if repeated six times or more, generate a picture in your mind (visualisation) which, if imbued with enough emotional charge, ie, passion and chi, will cause definite changes in your energy field [see *Psychic Egg* p. 54], which in turn will cause definite changes in your world along the lines you propose. Affirmations can take many forms, with one common principle: the statement is positive and in the present tense. The most basic form is the 'I am' variety, as in, 'I am beautiful, I am strong, I am healthy, I am capable of achieving anything I want'.

Then there is the 'I choose' kind, as in, 'I choose beauty, I choose strength, I choose health, I choose to achieve everything I want'.

There's the 'I deserve' sort, as in, 'I deserve beauty, I deserve to have what I want' etc.

And the 'I now manifest', more ordaining style, as in, 'I now manifest beauty in my life, I now manifest everything I want easily and effortlessly'.

You can mix em up, as in, 'I am strong and wise. I choose to use my strength and wisdom today to achieve something magnificent. I deserve something magnificent today. I now manifest a magnificent surprise'.

Speaking your affirmations out loud, especially in the presence of sympathetic others can enhance the magical force, which is how hymns, chants and incantations work.

Make up your own affirmations in any style you feel like, the more creative the better, as if the thing you're affirming is happening now. Avoid saying 'I will achieve an enormous amount today' as this defers the force to some imaginary time in the future, though obviously it would be better to say 'I will' than 'I won't', but best of all would be to say, 'I achieve an enormous amount today'.

Write down seventeen times: 'I have the power to manifest everything I want simply by affirming it to be so. As long as my affirmations are in accordance with the natural flow of what's going on, they work every time. When they don't work, it's because something bigger and better is coming my way. So be it.

Always end an affirmation session with a signing-off slogan such as 'so be it', 'so let it be', 'so must it be', or simply, 'that's how it is now'.

A hearty session of affirmations is the perfect antidote to a serious wobble attack and is a far more effective use of energy than worrying.

BLESSINGS AND CURSES

Because your words carry enormous power, it is important you use them wisely in your pronouncements to others.

Making pronouncements is like casting spells, as in spelling out your thought in word form.

You always have the choice between seeing a situation, yours or someone else's, in a positive or negative light. If a friend tells you their story and you choose to see it in a negative light and make a negative pronouncement based on that view, this is tantamount to cursing them. Medical doctors often do this inadvertently by mistakenly pronouncing someone incurable, ie, cursing them, thereby sabotaging the patient's recuperative power.

If, on the other hand, you choose to see that situation in a positive light and make your pronouncement accordingly, this is tantamount to blessing them.

So if someone comes to you complaining of their knee pain, telling them they'll never walk again is a curse, whereas telling them you see them hiking up a mountain in six months' time is a blessing. Obviously this would be stupid if they'd just had their lower leg amputated.

When people inadvertently curse you in this way, on account of their own negative bent, be sure to counter it with an affirmation of your own. For example, your friend says, 'You'll never achieve that', and rather than letting that negativity be the final command to the universe, you counter, 'I can achieve anything I choose to'.

May all curses be lifted from you now, and may you be blessed ten-thousand-fold with everything your heart desires.

PRAYiNG
On being a spiritual slut . . .

When you find yourself in one of those mystical/devotional frames of mind or in an emergency and you feel you want to pray, then pray. Don't ever be ashamed to pray or feel prevented by thinking yourself unworthy in any way. Fact is, whatever terrible thing you might have done, praying will always turn your energy around for the better.

Pray to whoever, whatever, and whenever you choose. Pray to the mountain, pray to the ancestors, pray to the Earth, pray to the Tao (but it won't listen!), pray to the Great Mother, pray to Jehovah, Allah, Buddha, Jesus, Lakshmi, Siva, pray to the Great Spirit, it makes no difference. You're free to deity-surf at your leisure. They will not penalise you on judgement day for being a spiritual slut. Praying is not for the benefit of the deity to whom you're praying, it's for you. Praying is like creating an envelope in which to send your heart's true desires to the main universal sorting office, which itself resides in your heart also.

There are no rules in this game. You don't have to believe in any particular god or goddess to pray. You don't have to follow traditional prayer forms. Praying isn't a religious affair, though it has been co-opted as such by various organisations we call religions. Praying is merely a device for realigning the mind, energy and passion of your local self with the mind, energy and passion of your universal (Great) self. When you pray, you're praying to the god or goddess within you. This has an effect on your energy field which in turn translates into a positive charge that makes something good happen. Praying

is another form of visualisation and is especially effective when used on someone else's behalf. Many warriors praying for the same thing in concert can move mountains. This is how teams work.

PATiENCE

if you have one wish, wish for everything to be exactly as it is. Then wait patiently for your wish to come true.

Waiting patiently for something good to occur is not a passive activity. Waiting patiently is an active state. With the full knowledge and faith that what's for you won't pass you by, and by breathing, relaxing and going with the spontaneous impulses which arise from within, you actively engage with the world, relishing every moment as it occurs, until in the fullness of time, that good thing you've been patiently waiting for will present itself in full manifest form before your very eyes.

You haven't wasted a single moment of your precious time here wishing it to be different. Patience means wishing everything to be exactly as it is, knowing full well, in the meantime, that according to the immutable law of yin and yang, things will change of themselves anyway and, if your original intention was clearly focused, they'll change along lines appropriate to your best interests. Patience, the quality of being a patient, is like entrusting yourself to the healer's hands, and letting them do what they're good at to help you get better.

Impatience, which affects us all at various times, is like telling the healer what to do. It doesn't work. Impatience is a form of self-pity, and is just another device for distracting yourself from what's actually happening in the present moment. If you wait impatiently for something good to happen, thinking that when that thing occurs your restless mind will find ease, you'll only find that as soon as the novelty value of that thing wears off you'll be left once again with restless stirrings trying to avoid the void [see *Fear of the Void* p. 77].

Waiting patiently, actively engaged with full conscious awareness in the present moment, with stillness in your centre in the midst of events, even angels will come to you, not to mention ordinary mortals, entirely of their own accord, to bring you everything you want, in the fullness of time, and may that time be a pleasant one.

Say fourteen times in a row, 'I am imbued with infinite patience, with infinite patience, I am imbued.'

PREPARATION
Prepare, prepare, prepare.

Always prepare for upcoming situations of importance by visualising, affirming or praying (if that's your tip at the time), for the outcome you want. Preparation will help you focus your intention and gather your chi into a concentrated force, so that you're able to deal effectively with that situation when it finally comes around.

A shorthand method to prepare for an event is to visualise the venue at which this event will occur and imagine it filled to the rafters with brilliant, all-pervasive, flushlight blue, special effects light, which touches all participants (even if it only involves you) and infects them with your positive spirit. This always produces a beneficial result for everyone, especially you, who will effectively have sent your spirit body on ahead to even the vibe [see Spirit Body *p. 57 and* Astral Travel *p. 140].*

On a more mundane level, preparation of body (hygiene, exercise and kit), equipment (pens, lap-tops, ropes, pulleys etc) and material (research, information, medicines etc) before any important event can also be used as a meditational opportunity to increase your psychic force in order to promote the best possible outcome. Like Japanese Tea Ceremonies or warriors sharpening swords before battles, mindful preparation sessions serve to focus your mind, body, chi and spirit into a concentrated point of intention. The ensuing force is as real as the point at the end of a sword that will penetrate and slice through the toughest resistance (with practice).

Ultimately, of course, a warrior is preparing for death, ie, that final crossing this time round, the biggest upcoming event of all, and may its upcomingness be in no hurry.

EXTRAORDINARY BUSINESS
ASTRAL TRAVEL
Cheaper and less polluting than air travel or public transport, less strenuous than riding a bicycle (but buy one anyway) and almost faster than light itself, astral travel, even with its strict zero baggage allowance, is fast catching on as the latest fad for a new breed of urban warrior.

I mean, think of all the fun you could have if you could do instant teleportation to any spot in the universe at any time in history. Well, you can or more true to say, you do already, mostly unawares, while you dream, and at the odd, unexpected psychic moment.

What this technique does is enhance your innate ability to send your spirit body instantaneously anywhere, anywhen, at will. Unfortunately the technology is not developed enough yet to allow you full physical teleportation, but we're working on it. However, this becomes inconsequential in the light of experiencing for yourself the immense delight of whooshing through the invisible cosmos in your very own personal spirit body, for deeds of derring-do, absent healings, love-making (yes, even that – but obviously only by consent, otherwise it's psychic rape), delivering messages and collecting important information. As well as the delight, think of the usefulness of being able to project into the future for purposes of visualisation, manifestation and information gathering. Imagine being able to send yourself to an important upcoming event ahead of time to smooth out the vibe and prepare your path.

Alternatively you can send yourself as you are now with all that you know, back in time to guide your past self through a difficult passage because, after all, who could guide you better, spooks and aliens notwithstanding.

And all you have to do is master scoopin' the loop so you've got a firm handle on your spirit body and then practise the following exercise:

You know how soldiers belly-crawl like snakes through the undergrowth (from time to time); well, the movement's like that, except you do it on your buttocks as you sit. First the right buttock moves forward, then the left, and you imagine that each forward movement propels you ridiculous amounts of distance at a time. But you don't actually move physically. You just imagine and feel you are, as you sit there with your eyes closed (after you've read this), casually scoopin' the loop, inside your psychic egg, an immortal spirit body boldly whizzing through the void.

You can go free-fall without predetermined destination and simply give your spirit body its head, which'll always land you up somewhere interesting, or you can select a point in time and space of your choice and make a bee-line. What you do when you get there is your business and beyond the scope of this Handbook, save to say that when you're operating on this level, you can do serious psychic and consequently physical damage to yourself and others by meddling where you're not welcome.

The return journey is most comfortably accomplished by circling in a broad sweep (sudden turns can be disorientating at first), until you can refix on the exact location of your physical body in time and space. As soon as you do this, you will be pulled back at psychic breakneck speed, which is a wicked rush, so remember to check your physical body out from the outside on your way back in, for an interesting perspective shift.

Once back in, settle yourself in the right direction (facing front) and take a moment for all parts of you to regroup fully. If in the process you do the odd scoopin' the loop, this will prevent any serious disorientation or distortion in your fundamental psychic shape.

If you find yourself suddenly snapped out of your astral journey by local Earth-plane disturbances, your spirit body will return instantly, and you'll arrive back in your physical form instantaneously if a little dishevelled, like when you've just been woken up from deep-dream sleep. This style of travel, once you get into it can become obsessive, so avoid using it as a distraction from things that need doing, or they'll call you 'Space Cake'. [See *Drug Culture – ketamin* p. 171]

COMiNG OUT THE BACK OF YOUR HEAD
On coming out the back of your head. Easy!

In extreme situations involving power struggles which could result in damage to your person or that of someone you wish to protect, whether psychic or physical in nature, when you wish to take possession of the situation in order to neutralise your opponent's force, and only in such cases, it is permissible to release your spirit body out the back of your head. This can cause a severe run on your power supply, leading to unpredictable after-surges and even total systems failure, and should therefore be trained slowly and patiently and not used as a toy in the presence of others though, if you're a power tripper, it will be tempting from time to time on account of the noticeable psychic advantage it gives you over whomever you're with. So use integrity.

At the back of your head, in the centre, where your neck joins your skull, is the rear door of the 'mysterious passageway', which leads directly to the cave of your original spirit, in the centre of your brain. Visualise this door opening (sliding doors work best) to allow egress for your spirit body. Now engage in nine mindful rounds of scoopin' the loop, or until you feel firmly ensconced in the shape of your spirit body. Breathing calmly with four-stage breathing, simply come out the back of your head, like a genie escaping the lamp, feeling yourself growing larger until you can look down at the crown of your own head. Look around you from this expanded perspective and focus your attention on an object, any object will do. Softly embrace this object within the psychic folds of your spirit until you have it completely engulfed, like throwing a net over a wild tiger. This should be practised with the eyes open.

If the need should arise, you can, with practice, perform this deft little manoeuvre on an opponent, and strange things will happen. Your opponent may even become your friend. Be sure to allow your spirit body back in through the same door afterwards otherwise it will seep back in through your nose and eyes, which can give you an itchy eye and runny nose condition for a few days.

Always rest and scoop some loop afterwards.

iNTUiTiON

Your intuition (literally tuition from within) will save you from potentially dangerous situations and prevent you making wrong turns, as long as you shut up and listen.

Situations produce vibrations. Negative, potentially harmful situations emit slow vibrations. Positive, potentially life-enhancing situations emit quick vibrations. As these vibrations impact on your energy field they produce either resonance or dissonance in your lower and middle tantiens, depending on your own vibratory rate at the time.

Exposure to slower vibrations will engender heavy, torpid feelings in your body and drain your psychic force. Exposure to quicker vibrations will engender light, vibrant feelings in your body, and charge your psychic force.

When your psychic force field is strong and your vibratory rate is fast, therefore, you will draw only positive situations to you. You will be automatically repelled by negative situations and 'accidents' will not happen. Your body will feel heavy and uncomfortable whenever you draw near danger. When your mind is quiet enough and your attention is on the moment, you will literally hear the dissonance in your belly and chest like an alarm bell going off, urging you from deep within your body to move in such and such a direction.

Always follow it.

At times these urges may come to you in the form of internally spoken dialogue with your higher self, spirit guide, guardian angel, alien intelligence, Harvey the Rabbit, or however you see the owner of that 'still, small voice within'. This form of dialogue can be entertaining and reassuring but is best not overindulged in as, in the extreme, it tends to lead to the loony-bin.

At times you may receive your messages from 'Indian' signs, such as slogans on passing trucks or cloud formations in the sky. This is also best kept in moderation, to avoid seeing signs in everything and becoming terribly confused. Just let it happen when it happens and don't try looking for it.

You can also use this vibratory barometer to assist you in making either/or choices. One option will make your body feel light, the other will make it feel heavy. Always go for the light.

FAILURE
There can be no death, there can be no failure, you have nothing to fear.

When you look at your life in terms of success and failure, you must remember that these terms are relative and not absolute. The criteria you judge by are spurious, subjective and based on limited perspective. If you judge success in terms of longevity, then death becomes the ultimate failure.

This is a most pessimistic view of your journey down the Great Thoroughfare; it means you are born to fail.

If, on the other hand, you judge success in terms of monetary wealth or status, you are destined too for ultimate failure, as you will lose both money and status at the final crossing.

If, however, you judge success in terms of the quality of time spent in full conscious awareness in present moment reality (the eternal moment), which can also include material wealth and longevity as by-products, you lose nothing at the moment of death and achieve the ultimate success of achieving an unbroken, silken thread of consciousness as you make the grand crossing.

Success is survival. Survival of your consciousness so far, that particular microcosmic access point to universal consciousness, peculiar only to you. And if you're reading this, you've done that. Congratulations, you've made it (so far), you're successful. In fact, when you consider the extreme unlikeliness of managing to take form like this, in such grand style, and furthermore to manifest all this magnificent scenery around you, not to mention the interesting company, and to sustain it even long enough to learn how to read, then I think double congratulations are in order.

In the light of having achieved this Herculean feat, the local disappointments you may suffer from time to time, such as losing money, love and other assorted forms of comfort, can hardly be considered failures. It would be more apt to call them signposts, lessons along the way to help you grow.

The best antidote to failure phobia is to love yourself. Love yourself whatever you're doing. No matter what. No exceptions. All the time. No matter how stupid, evil or ugly you think you are, love yourself thinking how stupid, evil and ugly you are.

Simply state, 'I love myself whatever I'm doing.' State this often.

When you get used to loving yourself whatever you're doing, you'll find it easier to love all others, whatever they're doing. Once you've got this, you have attained to buddhahood, at which point triple congratulations to you.

FEAR
The most important, essential thing for you, is to override your fear.

It is impossible to eradicate fear. This would be foolish anyway as it would divest you of a crucial ally. You need fear to keep you alive, both in emergencies and in day-to-day survival matters. Fear is not there to stop you. It's there to push you on in the right direction. It is not there to rule you, it's there to serve you.

Your fear prevents you from burning your hands in the oven but this does not prevent you from cooking food. To continue effectively on your path, your fear must be overridden. Overriding fear involves first acknowledging it and

COLLECTING

IMPORTANT

INFORMATION

then continuing in spite of it, quaking in your boots if need be. This trembling, open-hearted willingness to remain forever in your course, allowing the world to shape itself to completion around you, is true courage.

There are five basic kinds of fear, one of which will never be far from the surface. Closest to the surface is fear of starvation – not making a living.

One beneath that is fear of humiliation, ostracisation or banishment from tribe/support group – gaining a bad reputation.

Beneath that is fear of death.

Beneath that is fear of the after-life, hell, or being reborn into a horrible life as a common housefly trapped in a stuffy library, for example, ie, divine retribution.

Finally, at the deepest level, is fear of physical pain – discomfort along the way to reaching the death state.

Knowing these faces of fear will help you make friends with it. Making friends with fear will enhance your positive force. When you groove with the fear it transforms itself into excitement, hence the success of horror movies (adrenalin addiction).

Say, 'I am good friends with fear. We always get together when I'm in the mood for some excitement.'

DEATH
As a warrior, you're already dead.

Death, the final frontier, that dread final crossing into nobody knows what, is by all accounts an illusion. Nothing happens (and you can't prove that wrong either way). Sure, you leave your body, which can be painful, but once you've done that and the more self-confining layers of limiting mortal personality have dropped away, you merely find yourself where you always were when your awareness wasn't otherwise occupied in the social swirl of planetary life: sitting ensconced in the realms of eternity, watching as your dream-self habitually takes form, again and again, lifetime after lifetime.

This so-called death state (eternal life state) is where warriors go when they meditate, after thoughts subside and consciousness is still. It is said to be safe there and also much easier to work, as there are no longer any physical restrictions to obstruct you.

To take full advantage of this unconfined state, you'd be well advised to develop your relationship with your spirit body now, as this will be the vehicle that will contain and carry you there, the medium in which you'll continue your immortal existence, until the next time you forget and find yourself busting out of someone's womb (or egg!).

Reincarnation and dreams of after-life paradise notwithstanding, it is important to prepare for death, to feel willingness to let go gracefully at the appropriate moment, to shuffle off that coil with a straight heart as you return yet again to the great undifferentiated absolute.

The following contemplation will prepare you for hanging up those boots with style, with the immediate benefit of sizeably decreasing your overall fear levels.

Sitting comfortably, as you inhale, breathe in to the death state; simply be dead. As you exhale, breathe out into life, and regenerate the art-form you have created around you, ie, your life.

Every time you breathe in, completely withdraw your senses from Earth plane reality. Every time you breathe out, let your senses come out to merge with the entirety of creation.

This is heavy, hard-core meditation but, if practised with some regularity, will cause noticeable increases in enlightenment and general relaxation levels. When you feel at ease with your concept of death, practise being dead all the time, a mere phantasm, an illusion in people's minds. Being dead already means you cannot be killed or significantly harmed in any way, and thus have nothing to lose. Having nothing to lose, you have everything to gain, and whatever comes your way is pure bonus.

Note: it is contraindicated to make yourself physically dead before a full life-cycle (destiny) has been completed, as premature opening of the washing machine can cause ectoplasmic flooding on the floor. If you find yourself feeling suicidal, practising this contemplation may save you the trouble of the physical enactment, and save those left behind from having to mop up the floor.

BASiC REQUiREMENTS
Air, water, food, shelter, clothing, company and animal warmth (optional) are your first considerations. Once you've met these basic requirements, you can sit back with a bit of hope and watch the movie.

Assuming you have something relatively solid and stable to settle yourself on (a planet will do), the basic requirements you need are: air to breathe, water to drink, food to eat, a shelter to shield you from the elements, clothing to hide your naughty bits, company (invisible ie spiritual or otherwise) as a reference to stop you going nuts, and physical animal warmth ie love, especially in your formative years (optional but deprivation not highly recommended).

Whenever you find yourself in a tizz about not having enough material comfort in your life, run this check list. If all points get a tick, you're doing fine, and may your perspective return swiftly [see *Self-Pity* p. 110]. If any of the points get a cross, you'd better get busy or you die. It's that simple.

SHELTER

Choose your place of residence on the highest, most stable ground possible to soften the impact of sudden rises in sea level.

If your choice of geographical location is unrestricted, be up on a solid plateau, far from fault lines or volcanoes (active or dormant) in case our good Earth mother starts to rattle and hum, close to a source of fresh potable water, scarcity of which is fast becoming cause for sober consideration, and where you can grow enough of a varied crop of something edible to sustain you and/or be in proximity to others who are doing likewise. Try to locate where neighbours share the level of conscious awareness, and emit the kind of vibration you feel comfortable around.

If your life is currently more city-centre orientated, live as high up the nearest hill as possible for the air and close to open space, where your feet can touch naked earth/grass/seashore for your daily training session [see *Training* p. 18]. Avoid living close to power stations and pylons or living in areas that give you negative shudders [see *Intuition* p. 144]

Study some basic geomancy (feng shui), and observe basic principles of Earth-chi flow to avoid living over a diseased chi duct. Observe geomantic principles wherever possible in the decoration and arrangement of the interior, as this will augment your own chi flow and help smooth your way in the external world. Either avoid noisy places or keep a ready stock of ear plugs. Silence, ie freedom from engine noise, is fast becoming an endangered species, along with drinking water, and a warrior needs some silence from time to time, to receive the guidance from upstairs. Avoid living in damp, dark or draughty places.

Surround yourself with beauty as much as you can without getting obsessed.

Nothing is fixed. Everything is in a state of flux. Always be ready to move.

As a meditation on shelter, set sail on the sea of adventure, be without a permanent address for a while, sleep on couches or in palaces and go into full-on, free-fall Tao surfing mode for nine months.

Additionally, give spare change to homeless people whenever you can (and don't be mean).

AIR
All the air the world over is polluted.

Do not be fooled by idyllic scenes of purity. Concentrations of pollution are obviously worse the closer in you get to urban centres. Always breathe as deeply as possible, because the more poison you get in the more oxygen you get with it. Breathing shallowly won't protect you from the poison and will cause tension in your diaphragm, hindering your flow of chi.

So don't hold back. Breathe that filth in and transmute it with the power of your belief into life-sustaining chi. Take yourself to more 'unspoiled', less densely populated regions as frequently and regularly as possible, to get a few lungfuls of fresh stuff. Go outside early, when the cosmic chi is still clean and before the psychic as well as physical pollution has had too much chance to build up for the day.

Remember the air around you and value it like a fish does water. There is currently fourteen pounds per square inch of air pressure impacting on your body as you read this (unless you're in space).

WATER

Water for drinking, washing and sanitation is fast becoming a commodity to cherish, adequate supplies of which can no longer be taken for granted.

Thirty Chinese cities including Beijing are currently in the process of sinking due to excessive use of underground water. With China's ascending star in the world supremacy stakes, this situation will have consequences that could upset your breakfast one day (as in tea/coffee deficiency).

Water, the mother of all life, is the most tangible proof of magic and magical substances and is best not wasted by leaving taps or hoses on unnecessarily.

Give thanks every time you take a gulp, pray to it if you're that way inclined, and consider building up a small stock of water purification tablets for a non-rainy day.

FOOD

it's not the food that keeps you going, it's the chi in the food.

Although the food chain has a few rusty and broken links, don't let this deter you from enjoying a slap-up meal whenever you can. However, because of breaks in the chain causing distortions in the chi contained in food, living with a more or less dodgy stomach is fairly usual these days. Use your powers of visualisation to transmute everything you eat, including cornflakes, into first-class chi. Avoid dark meat (including lamb) as this tends to strain your liver and kidneys, which can cause arthritic symptoms, irritability and listlessness one or two days later. Avoid too much dairy intake as this increases mucous levels, damages your respiratory system and clogs up your energy field. Avoid fast and frozen food where possible because it has negative chi which will drain you within an hour. Avoid shellfish and go easy on fish altogether on account of rapidly rising sea pollution levels.

Go for a jolly colour balance of green, yellow and red food (eg cabbage, millet, peppers). Colour balancing is a quick and useful guide to yin-yang nutrition balance – don't eat too much blue!

The main thing is to eat food that has been prepared with love and is therefore invested with chi. When food has been invested with chi in the preparation, it doesn't matter so much whether it's fresh or organic, as the chi will be absorbed anyway, even if it's out of a tin.

Bless every mouthful you chew (ideally fifty chews per mouthful) by consciously choosing to extract the best quality chi from it.

Sit down when you eat, and let your entire focus be on eating, if possible. When simultaneously reading or engaging in spoken dialogue, let your primary focus be on digesting.

Avoid thinking problems over while you eat, as this will infect your chi with negativity.

Do not become obsessed by food quality. Vast numbers are starving every day. They wouldn't quibble about E numbers and preservatives, nor would you, so maintain perspective.

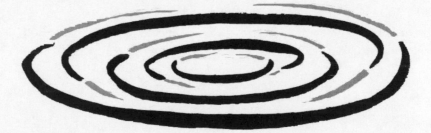

KIT

The primary function of your warrior kit is to protect your naked person from pernicious effects of the elements (wind, ie, draughts, water, ie, damp, heat, ie, sun, cold, ie, snow, ice, etc), ie, to provide an efficient layer of artificial fur (or feathers/scaly skin!) which will assist rather than hinder your body in its internal climate control function.

Effective layer management is therefore essential. Natural fibres, especially silk, allow chi to flow freely between you and the outside and should be worn as much as possible. However, synthetic fibre technology has advanced rapidly, especially in the realm of microfibres, and it is possible to have a relatively sweat-free, chi-conductive apparel experience in such-made togs. Advanced technology nylon outer shell (snow-board style) with a synthetic fleece lining is good for northern hemisphere winter months, and will offer efficient protection from wind.

Go without underwear whenever appropriate (but not in winter, wearing jeans on a bicycle, because it rubs) as this allows your sexual energy to flow more freely, rather than it getting caught up in your drawers [see *Hygiene* p. 157].

Wear as loose-fitting clothes as are fashionably practical as comfort is paramount. You need to be able to sit, stand, run, cycle, defend yourself, stretch, dance and work without your clothes exerting undue pressure on your vital or sexual organs. Don't, however, wear the crutch of your breeks (trousers/jeans/pants) too low, or you'll snag them on your bicycle seat when you dismount, which is most uncool and to be avoided in public places [see *Cool* p. 179].

Versatility of costume is also important, to enable you to fulfil all your various roles during a day, say riding your bike in foul weather to work, where you need to look 'presentable', then on to your martial arts class, on to a bar and on to a club (professional urban warrior agenda – remember to eat) with only one set of layers. Laws of social etiquette at the time of writing are relaxed enough to enable you to be appropriately attired for most situations in good quality work and sports wear.

Treat ties with caution, as these penile appendages are symbolic of being tied and enslaved and, though they are displayed proudly as alpha male markings, they are paradoxically symbols of disempowerment, not to mention plain useless and dangerous in a fight.

Footwear is like the tyres on a car, and must be of the highest quality and most intelligently built structure you can afford. Footwear technology has reached satisfactory enough levels to provide you with a most effective mobile base, especially in the realms of trainer culture. Always buy the top of the range whenever you can, as not only do these usually look better and therefore are more likely to be appropriate in more situations, but also because the more expensive shoe provides more effective ankle/instep support and heel/sole cushioning, which is vital for knee and hip happiness.

Go barefoot as often a possible [see *Your Feet* p. 37], because it's funky and helps you pick up messages from the ground, as well as massaging your reflex points in the soles to promote health in your vital organs.

Avoid excessive sweating in trainers and, if this should occur, wash said trainers in machine on cool.

Wearing trainers without socks causes fungus and stink-foot, which can be remedied by applying essential oil of lavender between your toes. Above all be sure your toes are not cramped, because cramped toes equates to cramped soul (sole).

Kit is also used to display tribal markings, the science/art of which has become highly sophisticated and convoluted. Choose the markings you display in such a way that you can cross easily from one tribe/country to another during the course of a day without having a single costume change.

Avoid wearing costumes that attract unnecessary attention in public places, as this nullifies your warrior invisibility privileges, and it's gauche! On the other hand, dress in as finely cut, well-made garments of the most magical hues and exotic fabrics as you can find, in order to contribute fully to the living art form of the street. You are an art form, but 'you' includes much more than your outer appearance, so do not become obsessed with clothes, no one's going to be looking at your shoes, and if they do, so what!

HYGIENE
Cleanliness is next to Taoliness.

When your body's dirty, your energy/chi will become dirty also. Being dirty reflects not wishing to let go of the past (however painful), as in clinging to the dust and grime of what's gone before. If you indulge in dirt, you're avoiding moving forwards. Washing on a daily basis (in busy, polluted urban centres, and on a bi-daily basis out of the city) is essential to maintain clean chi-flow, and keep your life moving on nicely, as in maintaining social popularity. This is best done in shower form, as baths waste too much water, and washing bits in a sink never really does it.

Transform the experience of washing into a meditation practice, by appreciating the magical properties of both water and the new present moment, leaving you ready as you towel off your privates to receive all kinds of gifts from the universe.

Brush your teeth at least twice a day and be careful with cotton sticks in your ears!

Maintain your kit in as pristine condition as you can, as clothing also gets old chi stuck, stalely, within in its folds.

Use natural soaps and shampoos whenever possible and avoid strong perfume, deodorant or cologne as first, it stinks, second, it messes up the aromatic balance of your energy field, and third, it sends false messages. Instead use subtle scents and essential oils, which tend to complement rather than mask your natural body smell.

Maintain your living space in as clean and dust-free a state as possible without becoming obsessive, as this will encourage healthy chi-flow.

Finally, avoid growing long beards (especially if you're a girl) as these can easily become tangled in bicycle wheels, get pulled hard in fights, and they harbour germs.

SLEEP

Sleeping is one of the most healing activities a warrior can partake in.

Your system will function adequately on four hours' sleep a day, with correct mental programming [see *Affirmations* p. 133, and *Intention* p. 64], however this may deplete your adrenalin levels after a while. Seven hours a night is enough to get your dreaming and self-healing done and, if commenced before the witching hour, twelve midnight, will be more potent.

Sleep-time is when your body regenerates itself and your energy is renewed. Sleep whenever you feel like, if possible, but do most of it in one hit. As well as healing your body, sleep heals your mind, outlook, alertness, attitude, mood. Your spirit receives information while you dream, often premonitionary in nature. This information can be accessed by writing your dreams down as soon as you wake up (this becomes easier in time). Your spirit also goes out to work during dream-time [see *Spirit Body* p. 57, and *Astral Travel* p. 140], memories of which (far and distant cosmic lands etc), can be accessed through meditation.

Sleep on your right side, coiled up like a dragon, so that the blood can spend the night in your liver, being washed, and away from your heart. Excess blood in your heart during sleep-time will give you crazy or alarming dreams.

Just before sleeping, consciously choose what kind of dream journeys you want, and how and when you wish to awaken, as in feeling bright-eyed and bushy-tailed at 7.23 am. Then, drawing your consciousness back into your cave of original spirit in the centre of your brain, look through the middle of your forehead, as if you have an extra (third) eye there. If you're successful in maintaining conscious awareness while descending deeper into sleep mode, you will at this stage be able to see the room you're sleeping in, through your forehead, lit much brighter than usual, just as if someone has left all the lights on in the room, with perhaps a few subtle changes. When this occurs, if you sink and relax and scoop some loop, you'll be able to follow your spirit body out on its secret adventures, just like Peter Pan or Wendy. If you want to float, fly or otherwise display powers of supernatural bent, simply see your hands drawn up to your magic forehead eye and examine them, front and back. This will put you in conscious control of the journey.

Insomnia results from having too much heart fire (adrenalin), which can be treated effectively by strategically applied acupuncture.

Sleeping disease arises from deficient yin or structive chi [see *Yin-Yang* p. 14], which is also effectively treated by acupuncture and herbs [see *Healing* p. 189].

HUMAN TOUCH
include human touch interludes as part of your daily agenda.

Touching other humans in warm and affectionate ways, and being touched by them likewise, is an essential factor in maintaining physical, emotional and psychic health. Chi is transmitted through touch (basis of Taoist healing). At the point of contact, chi-flow is accelerated, which is why it feels so good when someone touches you, especially with loving intention, as this softens the chi's texture.

Touch, as in shaking hands, hugging, massage, cuddling and healing, warms up your world and softens the tone of your interactions with others. Touching affectionately bridges communication gulfs far more effectively than talking, and comes highly recommended as an effective social device for spreading healthy chi and relaxed vibrations. Touch (with an average of four ounces of pressure), is also the most effective way to read someone's energy [see *Yielding and Sticking* p. 93].

Beware of physical contact with people of negative chi persuasion, such as practitioners of manipulative magic or those with vicious natures, as this will drain your own chi. If, after contact with someone, you feel suddenly cold, shivery or exhausted, it's likely you've just been tapped, in which case, shake the chi off your hands, like you would if you'd just dipped them in brackish water, and hold them under cold, running, fresh water, if possible, as a ritualistic gesture to yourself, signifying uncontaminated status confirmed, and do a psychic hoop and psychic egg visualisation.

TOOLS
You tool!

Keep your tools clean, ordered and in working condition. Your hands, your vehicles, musical instruments, decks, tunes, disks, computers, books, paints, film, hammers, saws, ropes and pulleys, basically everything you use for your work (money-earning or not) must be kept in ready-to-use status.

Your tools are an extension of you. Your chi and consciousness passes through them. Investing time in maintaining them is another form of meditation, a magical operation which will imbue your tools with power so that they serve you better. This also acts like a magnet drawing opportunities to you.

Visualise all your tools, including everything you use to keep you afloat (this may be all your possessions), and surround them all with soft, pink, special light.

MEDITATION – SHITTING AND PISSING
Never rush the process of evacuating your bowels or bladder except, of course, in an emergency.

Modern cultural conditioning, based as it was on the ethos of denial of nature (hence this global urban reality, where even birdsong is on the decline), has most of us trained to be ashamed of these two most essential 'empty trash' functions. But, in fact, a full release of bladder or bowel, at the appropriate time, is one of the greatest pleasures on Earth – and it's free, if you discount sewage and initial apparatus of set-up costs, toilet bowl and flush, etc. It is certainly nothing to be ashamed of and, in fact, provides a perfect opportunity for coming into full contact with nature – the Tao – in the midst of a busy urban day's doings.

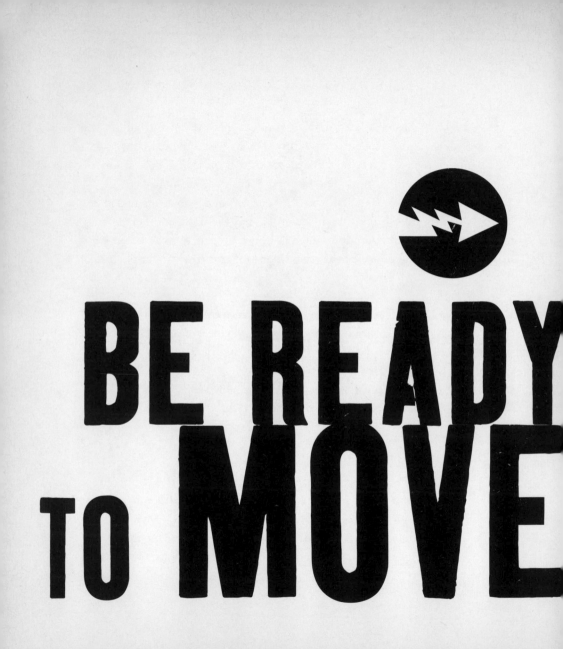

For the most effective (and potentially dangerous) bowel movement, squat over the bowl with your (bare) feet on the seat. If this is impractical, ensure that your back is as upright and relaxed as possible [see *Posture* p. 31], as cramping the intestines by leaning forward causes blockages and strain. Avoid straining your pelvic floor and specifically anal sphincter muscles by forcibly pushing out turds. Instead, relax, sink, breathe, centre and allow gravity to assist those rhythmic intestinal contractions, in simply letting go, just like giving birth, so faeces can fall of their own volition as they follow their quest for freedom on the open seas.

Same applies to urination, which should be a relaxed event for the bladder. It must be encouraged to release its load freely without having to fight resistance in your urethra caused by emotional tension (as in cystitis). For boy urinators, standing on tip-toes during the act, strengthens your kidneys. For girl urinators this technique should only be practised in open country on still days.

Urine and faeces are the wattle and mud of your past, and are best held on to for the minimum possible time. At the same time, they are strong reminders of your primal nature and must be honoured as such. While this does not mean going to the extremes of some fetishists with predilections along waste orientated lines, it is important to make the most of enjoying every piss and shit you do. Anyone who has lost these natural functions through bowel, bladder or kidney damage, or who is incontinent, will verify this: never take the empty-trash function of bladder or bowel for granted. Make full use of them everyday whenever able.

SEX
You're sexy!

To be an urban warrior, you've got to be sexy and feel sexy all the time. Your relationship with the world has to feel sexy. The way you engage on this planet has to be sexy. Your relationship with the divine realms – your spirit – has to be sexy. Everything you do has to be sexy, because sexy means connected, connected to the life-force, and when you're connected, you're authentic. This results automatically of itself when you practice this particular exercise:

Visualise a tubular channel starting in the sole of each foot, running up the inside of each leg to your perineum (between your anus and scrotum/vulva), and up to the tip of your penis/uterus.

From here it goes back down to the perineum, divides down the outside of each leg, and continues to the starting point in the centre of each sole.

As you inhale, feel as if the breath is entering the channel through the soles of your feet and travelling all the way up to your perineum, and upwards still to the penile/uterine tip, to fill your genitals.

As you exhale, feel the breath drop through the descending channel to the soles of your feet, ready for the next cycle.

Complete at least nine slow cycles, ending the last with the breath (chi) in your genital region.

This exercise will enhance your sexual energy flow. It should be practised along with scoopin' the loop and the psychic egg, as it creates a magnetic field which draws lovers like flies, and you may need a filter to sort the ladybugs from the mosquitoes.

Sexual energy is the most tangible example of chi. Sexual energy is also the most tangible example of the divine creative urge. Its elevated spiritual status is attested to by the fact it's so powerful you can even make new people with it. In other words, never be ashamed of your sexuality.

When your sexual energy is flowing, not only will you feel more spiritually and physically connected and on the pulse, but you'll also get laid more often.

This is because when your sexual energy flows freely throughout your body (not just your genitals), you'll be sexy, and when you're sexy, the whole world's sexy with you. Ask any commissioning editor, a TV programme has to be sexy to get the ratings, a book has to be sexy to be a bestseller, everything has to be sexy for people to want it, because sexy equates to godly.

Sexy results from sexual energy flowing freely through your system. This in turn brings confidence as the chi warms your heart, and gives you that touch of je ne sais quoi which turns those heads as you walk into that room.

Not only this, but it's also true to say that it's only possible to enjoy seriously satisfying sex when you're sexy.

Be sexy in all you do. Repeat this affirmation often: 'I am sexy. I am sexy. I am sexy. I am sexy. I am sexy. I am sexy. I am sexy. I am sexy. I am sexy. I am sexy. I am sexy. I am sexy. I am sexy. I am sexy. I am sexy. I am sexy. I am sexy. I am sexy. I am sexy.'

CONDOMS
Wearing a condom can be erotic.

Unless you're devoutly married or otherwise engaged in a fully committed coupled situation and stay that way for the rest of your sexually active time here, and are sure of testing negative, a good relationship with condoms is essential.

Those ancient viruses we've unleashed from the earth are highly intelligent and possessed of unlimited wanderlust. The transmission of the sexual variety, including Hiv, Aids, hepatitis B and C etc, and herpes is significantly halted by wearing a condom. It's that simple.

Yet there are vast numbers of people who, not believing they are mortal or susceptible, indulge in random coitus sans condom.

Often the reason for this, though masked in bravado, is fear. For the wearer, it's fear of losing his erection while putting on the condom, perhaps. Maybe he feels the condom emasculates him somehow or that it implies his penis is evil and should be kept apart during the intimacy of sex. Or he may fear losing his erection during penetration through decreased sensation.

For the recipient, there may be the fear of being considered prissy, paranoid or untrusting.

Now, by reframing the situation, doing a little perceptual shift, you could perform the action of condom-donning as if it were an erotic act, as if condoms were your particular fetish.

Imagine that wearing condoms is widely considered a highly erotic fetish and that to wear one is not only cool but sexy (after all fashions change according to mass shifts in perception) and visualise you or your partner putting one on with all the sensuous delicacy of an expert table dancer. Imagine the erection actually enhanced by that shimmering, shiny sheath. It's not such a far-fetched idea – after all, there are fashionable fetishes going around which are a lot more daft than that. Be sure to share this vision with all future sexual partners. Condoms are cool.

Finally, when all the shuddering and squirting is done and the erection begins to lose volume, be sure that one of you holds the condom around the base of the penis as you withdraw, to prevent it coming off inside.

TRANSPORT

The most cost-effective, energy-efficient, pollution-free form of transporting yourself from place to place in time and space is by using your own legs, especially your quadriceps (front thigh muscles) to propel your feet in a walking, running, cross-country skiing, or peddling, as in cycling, motion, unless you live on water, in which case use biceps for rowing or swimming.

Any other method (crawling or astral travel notwithstanding) will involve the energy of either animals (horses, reindeers or huskies, etc) or other people (sedan chairs, rickshaws, solar/water/battery powered vehicles, or fossil fuel-burning combustion engine vehicles). Animal-drawn vehicles, sedan chairs and rickshaws are largely impractical these days, solar/water/battery powered vehicles are still, at the time of writing, largely unavailable and fossil-fuel-burning vehicles (cars, trucks, buses, trains, boats, ships and planes) require inordinate portions of human energy and resources (in the design, financing, administration, raw material facilitation, manufacture, distribution, road-building, etc). Additionally, and more importantly, the burning of fossil fuels to power combustion engines, itself requiring vast human resources in the mining, refining and distribution thereof, happens to be rapidly destroying the air we depend on for our immediate survival. In other words, the enormous volume of fossil fuel-burning traffic on the world's roads, flight paths and sea lanes in any one day, today for instance, is polluting us out of existence. So though we're designing the cutest, sleekest vehicles (toys), there may only be the spiders left to drive them.

Every time you go from place to place by any other method than moving your own muscular/skeletal system, you are therefore contributing significantly to your own demise, not to mention mine.

Using public transport systems helps to reduce this effect, and is a good way to enjoy human contact without getting involved, but is inadvisable during rush-hour except where unavoidable.

Walking, cycling and running (with use of backpack for work togs), ie, self-propelled transportation, does not poison the air or speed your demise (as long as you stay alert). On the contrary, it may actually prolong your life on account of the muscular, respiratory and cardio-vascular exercise, not to mention the pleasant altered state of mind engendered.

If you're fortunate enough to have use of your limbs, use them for transportation as often as possible. Obviously, until solar/water/whatever powered vehicles are widely available, you will still be using combusters to expedite various trips. A hang-glider won't get you across the Atlantic or Pacific Ocean too efficiently, and you can't usually move house on a bicycle, but you will enhance your life experience significantly and contribute to a reduction of atmospheric poison every time you choose self-propelled over fossil-fuelled. Not only this, but you largely free yourself from the restrictions of massed movement of people – traffic jams – and thus feel more empowered.

In plain terms, ride a bicycle. Always utilise your psychic shielding function [see Psychic Egg *p. 54] and/or pray for protection [see* Praying *p. 136] before and during all transit operations.*

iNTERNATiONAL TRAVEL
As a warrior you are free to roam where you will, the road may appear to be somewhat obstructed from time to time, but don't let that deter you.
Your travelling kit/disguise for passing through airports/border patrols is best kept as discreet as possible and must fall broadly into categories currently accepted as unremarkable, such as business person, happy tourist or

outdoorsie backpacker, so as not to draw undue attention from customs officials and the like. Not to suggest that you may be actively engaged in illegal pursuits, but arousing suspicion by being too creative in your attire, therefore appearing 'out of the norm', can get you stopped/searched/refused entry, which will obstruct your path, slow your progress and drain your energy.

Always ensure your psychic shield is fully functional during travel of any kind to increase your invisibility factor, and keep your travelling papers (passport, tickets, etc) and money safely sequestered about your person at all times.

Wherever you go, tread lightly, contain your chi, and approach everyone you encounter with modesty and grace [see *Manners* p. 200].

In treading lightly, only carry as much baggage as you can manage yourself or are willing to take responsibility for, ie, pay a porter. If you lumber someone else with your baggage, without their whole-hearted enthusiasm, you'll be leaking chi and losing friends.

Wherever you travel, assume you're being guided by higher self/spirit body/the Tao in order to spread your healing chi whatever the superficial reason for your trip. As such, you are an ambassador, and are therefore granted immunity, so if you're meant to be somewhere, don't be deterred by immigration restrictions, you will be guided on how to gain entry and remain there. Trust that.

Also remember that the longest, most exotic journey you can imagine to anywhere on the face of the globe, is a mere fly in the eye compared to the journey you're actually making right now, as this planet hurtles through deepest space at 66,000 miles per hour.

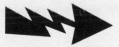

INTERFACING WiTH THE iNFRASTRUCTURE

Behind every stratum and facet of the infrastructure, however vast, complex and convoluted it may appear, are people.

The global infrastructure consists of various nation states, each controlled by a government, 'democratically' elected or otherwise, by the use of laws upheld by threat of brute force – police and/or military. The mechanics of daily life are regulated by civil services (mostly unelected but under control of government) which spread to local level.

These sectors (the nation states) are joined in various alliances or groupings by trade/military links, usually in opposition to one another, though alliances continuously shift and transmogrify. The status quo is regulated by international laws and agreements upheld by threat of brute force (nuclear/chemical/biological/dynamite etc).

These trade/military links are serviced mostly by multi-national corporations/conglomerates, who control the movement of resources via communications, shipping, transportation, manufacture, finance and distribution. The results of all this activity then filter down to local level, enabling you (the punter) to buy those tampons you just saw advertised on TV, at your local shopping mall or corner shop, without getting mugged, raped or terrorised.

And other than the fact that our atmosphere is polluted, water contaminated, food chain diseased, our lives threatened by terrorism, Fascism, fundamentalism, advanced chemical, nuclear and biological poison, and our minds largely controlled by the media, ie, other people, you could say the infrastructure is working out fairly well.

In fact, I'd say it's a miracle we're all still here at all. And that's the miracle to go with. In so doing, however, it is important to keep your doings within the legalities of the prevailing infrastructure, if you wish to ensure optimum freedom of passage. Nevertheless, it's helpful to be on good terms with a proficient and friendly lawyer, preferably adept at both civil and criminal law, for the odd occasion you may fall foul.

When dealing with police or military, use your psychic shield, and always remember your manners, as they are also people with feelings just like you, who will, on account of superior back-up, usually prevail in any contretemps or set-to.

That's the point. All people are ultimately governed by their spirits, no matter how crude or thuggish they be, and at the level of spirit, we, all people, are connected (Great Spirit). This is why it can often be more effective to meditate than demonstrate for infrastructural change, if that's your bent or desire.

See yourself in the midst of a vast psychic grid, comprised of lines of special-effects light, which psychically link your spirit body to the spirit body of every other person on the planet (or in the entire universe if you're feeling expansive), through the three tantien system.

Visualise yourself linking up to all the people involved in managing the global infrastructure, one by one, like millions of lights going on. With the belief that you can radiate the quality of compassionate wisdom ie peace and love, let this quality pour forth from your heart and touch everyone with a moment of divine sanity. This is an effective way to campaign for world peace.

DRUG CULTURE
Drugs, drugs, drugs

At the time of writing most of the substances mentioned in the by no means exhaustive list below are illegal in most countries and, though I am not advocating their use and, in most cases, would discourage it other than for medical or religious purposes, if you should find yourself with one or more coursing through your arteries, here are some factors to consider. (I've written this as the healer who's witnessed enough 'legal' and 'illegal' drug tragedies, rather than as the naughty taoist rascal, so you might find the tone unnaturally unromantic.)

Hash, grass (including hydroponically grown skunk), ie, THC, is the mild analgesic which Queen Victoria herself used to alleviate dismenorrhea (period pains) and which helps soften outside-world impact on your system. THC tends to scatter your chi, which can hinder concentration and therefore short-term memory, in return for magicking up your reality for an hour or so.

While true that THC can enhance your creative concentration, especially around music and visual arts, high doses may occasionally bring on paranoia attacks and prolonged use can lead to psychosis as in skunk psychosis, which in rare cases, when psychic structure is not adequately formed, can tip you into loony land on a long-term basis.

It's vital to balance THC intake with ample intelligent exercise like tai chi, running or yoga to keep the organs from stagnating, and to practise centring devices described in the Handbook to keep you focused in the moment. Being mashed in a soppy stoned heap weakens your psychic shield and may leave you unnecessarily vulnerable to danger, so practise psychic shielding techniques.

There is nothing sacrilegious about meditating or centring in a mindful way while intoxicated. Better this than wasting the time worrying. Main thing is to not let it make you lazy, crazy, or in any way prevent you from your path.

MDMA (E), the medicine that chilled a nation, is difficult to come by in pure form and is usually only available diluted, often cut with speed, heroin and/or other even more sinister components which may seriously damage your person.

While an effective emotional painkiller and dance enhancer, E weakens your kidneys, stresses your liver and heart and consequently lowers your immune response. Originally popular amongst the experimental therapy fraternity, it was never intended for use as a mass sacrament, as maintaining stable body temperature is essential for kidney balance, and this cannot be done effectively in the comings and goings of a hot club, even though it may feel good at the time.

Massage your kidneys well before, during and after ingestion, using your fists in a circling motion.

Fast for eight hours beforehand, eating only fruit and drinking water to help take the strain off your liver. Avoid mixing with alcohol, as this creates excess pressure on both liver and kidneys.

Be prepared for midweek blues, and if these should arise, use them positively to learn more about yourself.

As an alternative, Herbal Es rely mostly on ephedra (ephedrin) for psychotropic effect, which may clog your lungs with mucous and can make you melancholic. Though these are natural, the herbs used are strong and will seriously destabilise your system if used frequently.

Pay close attention to dependency patterns, as prolonged use of euphoric enhancers will produce long-term depression of all physical and psychic functions. If this occurs, get help from a strong healer (acupuncture is highly effective for this).

Remember to keep breathing and relaxing if you take a dodgy E .

Acid (LSD), in tab or dot form, is usually sold in manageable enough doses for you not to go round jumping out of windows. However, apart from fairly mild hallucinations, along the colour-enhancement line, audio distortions and time-stretch/shrink illusions, acid is little more than a cheap thrill and dance enhancer, its religious significance having been largely lost in the colourful mists of the late sixties and seventies, though its contribution as a creative laxative to the shape and coloration of our current culture has been both crucial and far-reaching.

Tripping will weaken your kidneys so do for them as you would for E. Eating an orange or drinking orange juice will help neutralise the trip if it's getting too much or going on too long. If you feel imminent loss of sanity, bring yourself back into your body, by breathing and gently pummelling on your chest like Tarzan for a minute or so. Scoop a lot of loop, centre yourself, and prepare yourself for moments of disorientation in the following days.

Ketamin (aka Special K) is a strong anaesthetic, conventionally used for child and pet surgery which, if ingested in sufficient quantities, will give you an enforced out-of- body, astral journey of such velocity you will either return with the knowledge of the gods/goddesses or the delusions of a mad person. Prolonged use can play havoc with your urinary-genital system, in some cases making it almost impossible to urinate for days on end, significantly weaken your liver, damage your vocal chords and depress your immune response. Enforced astral travel [see Astral Travel, p. 140) to where is, to all intents and purposes, the realms of death (eternal life), if experienced often enough will lead to morbidity and, in more extreme cases, suicide. This death-attraction state will occur over time even on the lower doses usually taken in social situations.

It is always advisable to counterbalance Ketamin flights with some serious acupunctural applications. Preferably 'fly' in the company of someone with enough presence of mind and warrior ability to look after you. Dedicated meditation practice is effective for preventing total post-flight disorientation and affirmations such as 'I choose to stay alive', can be effective mid-flight.

As with acid, bringing yourself back into your body by doing Tarzan pummelling on your chest can help in major crises.

Mushrooms, though sort of 'unillegal' in most places, are nevertheless potent medicine, and can occasionally cause sudden death from heartattack, even those sweet little liberty caps. Treat all 'shrooms with great respect, being the vision-giving, fairy medicine of the followers of the old ways that they are, and restrict use to daytime spiritual recreation in natural environments during daylight hours. Counter their effects on liver and kidneys by fasting, massage and acupuncture as with all other hallucinogenics.

Iahuasca (vine of the soul), Peyote buttons and mescalin are mostly confined to ritualistic, religious use among controlled situation groups (mostly native American), and are not at the time of writing wide-scale street drugs. However 2CB, an MDMA derivative, the synthetic version of mescalin, is becoming more readily available. Like acid, this is a vision enhancer and is usually taken as part of a cocktail with E. There is possibility of long-term memory damage, depression from regular use, and a distinct hardening of attitude. Can also cause temporary joint stiffness and pain, resulting from pressure on the kidneys.

Cocaine is an analgesic. Sniffing or smoking it closes your heart centre, which can make you abrasive to be around. As the heart centre is the conduit for brotherly/sisterly love, prolonged use of coke can in time isolate you and mess up your social life and career. It is highly habit-forming and, just like nicotine, is difficult to drop from your repertoire. Addiction is often accompanied by telling lies to those who love you, which weakens your integrity and clouds your decision-making processes. Smoking it in extreme crack form rapidly turns you into a dangerous zombie, and quickly reduces all possibilities of redeeming your warrior status. If ever there was a little devil that came in white powder form, coke is it. If you've had a line, be sure to pay extra attention to opening your heart centre.

Heroin, like morphine and other opiates, is an analgesic often appealing to more sensitive, creative folk, ingestion of which threatens ongoing maintenance of warrior status. Like cocaine, opiates are powerful and can destroy you more rapidly than necessary. Though some addicts, usually those with private incomes, can maintain a semblance of warriorhood by regulating doses over a prolonged period, it may well all end in tears. Conversely ex-addicts often reinvent themselves and go on to achieve true greatness. An effective counterbalance to opiates and cocaine is abstention. When this is difficult, visit a powerful healer [see Healing p. 189].

Speed (aka Whizz) is dirty. It will keep you going when necessary, but leave you feeling soiled the next day. It puts strain on the liver, which makes you depressed afterwards and gives you spots. Ice, the extreme form, is merely a big-dipper suicide trip, and is probably best avoided.

Sedatives, tranquillisers, sleeping pills and muscle relaxers (often used by E-heads, coke heads and trippers to help them catch the sleepy train) are highly habit-forming, and their use is best restricted to emergencies, like funerals of closest kin, as long-term use will flatten liver chi and depress your animal spirit.

Alcohol is an analgesic with social and emotional laxative properties, prolonged and extreme use of which will cause you to leak chi and what-have-you all over the place. Drinking can make you stupid and potentially violent. Alcohol weakens your kidneys, liver and spleen when taken in excess, and intake must be regulated at all times to preserve fully-functional, active warrior status.

Nicotine, active ingredient of the sacred tobacco plant, is a mild adrenalin stimulator, which is ingested in the modern cigarette smoking ritual as a way to mildly distract from restlessness or anxiety and to stave off boredom and loneliness. Smoking affects mostly liver, lungs and heart. This effect can be partly counterbalanced by regular aerobic exercise (walking, running, cycling) and regular relaxing/focusing exercise (tai chi, yoga etc).

Coffee is a fairly potent quick-hit stimulant, which gives the adrenals a little kick, but weakens them at the same time. When you drink coffee, it'll be more difficult to sink, so pay more attention to relaxing/sinking procedures. Tea is a milder, slightly less kidney-abrasive stimulant, but you can only really get a good cup in the UK (don't know why – maybe it's the water).

The ingestion of stimulants has always been an integral part of human experience. If however you should find yourself habituated to one or more, and you wish to free yourself, focus not on giving up, because that just keeps reminding you of the substance you're trying to forget. Instead, focus on developing positive activities, like tai chi, meditation, healing, etc. Focus on building the positive and the negative will take care of itself (or it won't – but at least you won't be such a drag to be around. You'll stop when you stop).

Whatever substance you may ingest, make a contract with yourself not to get so out of it you can no longer control your bodily functions, including walking, defending yourself and running away from danger, unless there is someone fully willing to look after you, but then you owe them one.

CULTS, GURUS, MASTERS/MISTRESSES

Always be wary of other people's trips. You contain the blueprint in your own circuitry which, when activated, will trigger all the information you need for your enlightenment and successful passage through.

While it's true that the trigger can often come through other people, ie, teachers, they are only reminding you, and not giving you anything that wasn't already contained in your original blueprint.

No one knows the answer any more than you do. There is no question in the first place, you just think there is. When it comes down to it, there's no one there to ask it anyway. The Tao carries all knowledge and at your core, that's what you'll find.

Obviously you need guidance from those more experienced, and must take optimum advantage of it when it comes your way, but this guidance, if accurate, will only help you deepen in your own innate knowledge of Tao. All any true teacher can do is guide you along your own self-determined path.

Anyone who tries convincing you that the only way to enlightenment is through them is a con artist, however grand or convincingly clear-eyed and holy they may appear.

Approach all teachers with absolute respect, learn whatever you can from everyone, let your process of self-discovery be triggered and retriggered by every encounter, but don't surrender your path to anyone, especially someone who calls themselves a master/mistress/guru/avatar/incarnation of deity.

A true master, someone who has learned to still their mind enough to be living consciously from the deepest stratum of reality, ie, the Tao, is discreet and will never call themselves master, for that would be courting disaster.

Swearing allegiance to someone who does guru-ing for a living (mass-hypnosis/cult running) is giving your warrior power away. Never do that. If you have done so and currently find yourself enmeshed in a cult of any sort, and wish to retrieve your personal power, exercise your right to use the break-off clause, face the demons and guard-dogs and get the hell out of there. As a warrior, your path is self-determining. Sure, chant with them, learn with them, meditate with them, get shakti (chi) from them, respect them, but don't follow them. Follow your own Tao.

Say nine times immediately, 'I only follow my own path. I am free to do whatever I choose. My choices are life-enhancing for everyone.'

Now say, 'I no longer blindly repeat the words others tell me to.' (!!!)

COOL
Cool

Being cool, the innate ability to respond appropriately in every situation, requires literally maintaining your chi at a cool enough temperature that it doesn't rush upwards through your chest and head (heat rises) and cloud your vision, choice-making faculties, personality functions and physical actions. Containing your chi in your belly allows your heart to be steady, so you don't get over-excited or panicked, and your head to be clear, so you can see the best move to make next and not lose the plot.

When you contain the chi in your lower tantien your movements will appear graceful [see *Stealth* p.98], and you will rarely be given to blathering or idle chit chat. Having a still, bluster-free mind gives you an air of natural modesty, which enables you to be sensitive to the vibrations of others and to interpret their chi. Interpreting the chi of others gives you command of every situation. Being in command allows you clear sight of the best of what's on offer around you at any time. Hence you'll choose the appropriate costume for every role you play, the appropriate mode of transportation, and the appropriate music to wobble your soundwaves just so, as you go. In short, contain your chi with dignity [see *Posture* p. 31], and you'll be cool.

Being cool does not preclude radiating warmth, ie, love. That would be being dull. Dull is no good (we don't talk to you) and must be avoided. Being cool is colourful because being cool is being a channel for the zeitgeist, ie, spirit or Tao, which is a multi-hued and sexy affair [see *Sex* p. 164].

One of the most important aspects of the being-cool experience is the inevitable occasional occurrence of a totally-uncool-attack. At these times, when you lose control of your chi and you make a fool of yourself, simply immerse yourself in embarrassment, which is the closest thing to bliss, in terms of valid altered states, and receive the experience as a signpost to point you back to cool.

The main trick with cool is to know it's cool to be a fool.

COMiNG OUT OF THE SYSTEM
However solid it may appear, there is no system.

Just billions of people, joining up at least five days a week to engage in habitual interactions, the form and terms of which have been previously agreed upon, but which are subject to change as things progress and which, one way or another, lead to pollution in the atmosphere and sewage in the sea.

Hence by group consensus, you have traffic jams at rush hour, globally, every morning and every evening, and people the world over believing in the power of money. A minority regulate the status quo of this conundrum and the majority goes along. This is normal and results from the inefficient use of imagination on the part of the individual.

As a warrior, however, you have the freedom to choose your own path and, as long as you don't get too attached to home, status and possessions, will be free to exercise that choice whichever regime is in power. In other words, just because everyone else is doing it, doesn't mean you have to too. Just because the majority live their lives a certain way, doing traffic jams twice a day, doesn't mean that's the right way for you. In fact, if you examine the mess made by the majority over the years, it's a safe bet to say that if you do the opposite you'll be on the right path.

This is not to advocate anarchy or chaos. It is simply to say that if you live from your imperishable core, in harmony with your authentic self, you will be following your own path/Tao, and not necessarily the path everyone else seems to be following. You will then automatically find yourself choosing work [see *Your Life's Work* p. 185] and play situations mostly out of the nine to five context, and mostly find yourself riding your bicycle or, if you must, driving your car to work, against the traffic.

You are an individual, literally one who is not divided. This means that to be authentic and live an authentic life you must be clearly focused on a single path, which means being focused on a single point. When you are thus centred, you see that there is no system, just lots of individuals playing in the playground. There is no system to come out of or rebel against. You simply play how you choose.

This is no less valid when living under the jurisdiction of a totalitarian regime, you just have to be more discreet about it. A warrior is always free.

A quick cut to seeing through the illusion of systems is to do the upside-down contemplation:

You have always assumed that the sky is up and the ground is down. This is based on the now defunct flat earth theory. As we are actually on a globe, it is only possible to say that the sky is further out away from the Earth's centre, and the ground is further in towards the centre, relative to where you're standing. This being so, it is perfectly acceptable to replace this nonsense of sky-up and ground-down with its opposite nonsense of ground-up and sky-down.

Just like a bat hanging 'upside down', you imagine that the ground you're hanging off is up, and the sky into which your head is hanging down, is down. Look up to the floor and down to the ceiling. The tree-tops are reaching down into the sky. Birds fly down there, and planes go really deep.

Practise this lying, sitting or standing still and then take it out for a walk or run. This visualisation is powerful and can make you throw up if you overdo it on a full stomach. As well as helping you to see through the apparent system in general, mastering the upside-down contemplation is effective in high-stress situations like courtroom dramas, and other such instances where the 'system' illusion is strong. A few moments of upside down will concentrate your chi and spirit. It's also wicked in a headstand.

For more complete coming-outness, don't use credit cards and only borrow money from friends.

SUPPORT SYSTEM – GLOBAL TRiBE
A warrior cannot live in isolation.

It's time to come out of isolation and join with all the other members of the global tribe, accept your interdependence, pool your resources and move on to the next part of the story, whatever that is.

Trouble is, a vast number of your global brethren/sistren will often both get on your nerves and in your way from time to time.

So you work on yourself to find your own centre and points of reference, gather yourself, gird your loins and come out to play, skilfully negotiating your way through the obstacles and irritations thrown up by aforementioned tribe members. This is because you have learned as a warrior that you cannot live in independent isolation, unless you live as a mountain-cave-hermit on nothing but air, and even that is affected by everyone else. Instead, you learn to live in healthy interdependence with everyone else on the planet. This requires you trust that everyone involved is playing their appropriate role in the drama to the best of their ability at the time, however much it looks like they're fucking it up sometimes.

In so doing, you start to notice the perfection in everyone you meet. Perfection in the sense that everyone is acting out their role to perfection, even if that role of someone who is perfectly engaged in getting on your nerves or apparently obstructing your path.

Once you see the perfection in everyone, you tend to draw, by the immutable law of affinity, those who are specifically perfect for you at this time.

If you then look around you with clear eyes, you will notice people in your immediate circle who are willing, potentially and actually, to engage in a mutual support scenario. These people may or may not have any connection to members of your blood-family, but they are for sure members of your warrior family. Treat them well, in accordance with your generous nature and they'll do likewise. Look after the members of your warrior family and they'll look after you. Expect nothing, however, and you won't be disappointed. Everyone, even the most magnificent warrior, will get on your nerves and in your way from time to time, at which times you negotiate or give them space.

Say, 'I have clear vision. I have strength. I know what I'm doing, and no one or nothing can stop me.' And, 'I live in healthy interdependence with all creation.' And, 'I give and receive love freely.' And, 'People like to help me.'

PEOPLE SURFiNG
You have no obligation to become or remain entangled in someone else's life story.

There are many, however, who, for misguided reasons of their own, will attempt to enmesh you by hypnotic suggestion and emotional manipulation. You are always free to spend your time as you wish, within the current framework of your reality [see *Reality and Belief* p. 86], ie, if you're in prison or living under a totalitarian regime, for example, your available sphere of influence and activity will appear more limited.

This means that while you may love everyone who comes into your orbit with the compassion of a buddha, you must not attach yourself to anyone else's story. You enter Earth Phase as an individual with an individual story, and you leave it in the same way. You are free to share that story with other individuals as often as you like, but it's still your story. Other individuals are free to share theirs with you likewise. This allows a free flow of energy/love between you based on your authentic self rather than your ideal/well-behaved self. And though there will be pain on letting go when those times of orbit expansion occur, this must not stop you moving on when the mystery and adventure of the Great Thoroughfare beckons.

In other words you are free to people surf. Always observing correct protocol [see *Manners* p. 200], and coming from your authentic self, you actively engage in the free sharing of chi/love/information, in whichever ways are most appropriate or comfortable for you, with whomever you want, for however long you want (by mutual consent). And when you've had enough for the time being, you're always free to move on, being sure to keep the links intact so you can come back when you choose.

Everyone on this planet is your sister or brother, all walking along together down the Great Thoroughfare, holding hands, helping each other into the unknown; some a little further ahead guiding the ones a little further behind.

(There's lots of chi/love/information to be shared, and there may not be lots of time, so get surfin'.)

YOUR LiFE'S WORK
Whatever you do for a living, your life's work is to heal yourself.

Healing means to make whole, as in round yourself into a fully functioning, completely interactive, multi-media, poly-dimensional living art form, which expresses the unique essence of who you are in your imperishable core, for the enjoyment, entertainment and education, ie, enrichment of others. The wholeness you display teaches others by example, who are then inspired to find wholeness for themselves.

Wholeness or healing spreads through all your relationships like a light which makes the world warmer and kinder for everyone. In other words, by healing yourself, you heal everyone around you. By delivering/ broadcasting the particular message of who you are, you are bringing your unique gift to the world, your unique brand of love, wisdom and chi, like a flower unfolding its Divine magic, opening for all the world to enjoy and benefit from.

No matter whether you work at the supermarket checkout, the Stock Exchange, the circus or the clinic for distressed artists, your real work behind the scenes is to heal yourself and everyone you encounter, in whatever guise, with your love, energy and wisdom during the course of a normal day's doings. You don't have to work as a healer to heal people. You can do it while driving a cab, for example. It's all down to radiating a positive personal atmosphere [see *Blessings and Curses* p. 135].

However, if you feel drawn to the path of mastering the five excellences mentioned next, this will provide an excellent context in which to frame your healing work.

If you follow the path of your own healing, every kind of opportunity you need to help you fully express yourself will open up to you of itself.

Say seven times very quickly, 'I now express the full unadulterated beauty of who I am, and share it with everyone in my world. I let it come through everything I do, no matter how trivial or mundane. That's how I alleviate the suffering of others and fulfil my life's work.'

GRAFFiTi
Writing's on the wall.

The magnificent pieces which adorn our train carriages, public walls and bridges are possibly the most poignant artistic statements of our times. Given freely, at great personal risk to the artist, they personalise and colourate an otherwise bland cityscape. 'Writing' expresses a global language, which points to the need for us to recognise and honour the individual, ie, the undividable spirit within each of us. The tag, denoting the identity of the individual artist or crew, represents the alter-ego, or higher self.

Writing, however, is mostly illegal, except in more enlightened enclaves like Amsterdam and I in no way wish to encourage you in this pursuit. Though if you find yourself addicted to this particular form of adrenalin addiction, you would be well advised to avoid detection by members of various law enforcement agencies. Obviously it is important to choose your site prudently, and to refrain from defacing private property. Your intention must be to positively enhance the experience of life for others. This will attract positive energy to you, and stack your credit with the spiritual powers that be (guardian angels and the like), who will then be more well disposed to watching over you while you work.

Always pray for protection, make use of full psychic shielding facilities and carry a 24-hour contact number of a proficient criminal lawyer. Although there is no substitute for the purity of authentic adrenalised street art, you can easily progress along your creative path by transferring to canvas [see *Career - The Five Excellences*, p. 187].

CAREER — THE FiVE EXCELLENCES
The five excellences: a magnificent career opportunity for those with nothing better to do.

Traditionally, the Taoist warrior would aspire to becoming master/mistress of the five excellences. These are the arts of self-defence or pugilism (knock 'm down), medicine or healing (fix 'm back up), meditation or magical operations (collect yourself after all that fighting and fixing), music or song (without which what would be the point?) and poetry or calligraphy (ability to communicate with words or mesmerise). Martial, medical, magical, musical and mesmerising are the five excellences.

The warrior mastering these arts will enjoy a healthy, full, balanced life and will always be able to make a living, ie, survive, nay thrive, even in the event of cataclysmic, social, political, economic, environmental or geological disruption, and enjoy a rich social life.

In plain terms, learn a martial art (tai chi, xing yi and pa kua come highly recommended) to give you protection, alertness, chi control, fitness and health.

Learn a healing art, such as acupuncture, massage, bone setting or chi-transference, so you can take care of those around you. Learn to meditate for inner peace and clarity, and to do magic to shape new worlds with. Learn to play an instrument, sing, dance, act, juggle, story-tell, or any other performable or visual art so you can entertain the troops and keep their spirits high, in other words, lead groups. Learn to communicate clearly in words, written or spoken so you can teach others (martial arts, medicine, mediation, music and mesmerising).

In this way you'll always have something to offer for trade. You'll always be given a roof over your head and food in y' belly and, who knows, you may even become a star (or a barefoot doctor).

HEALING
Did you get the healing?

You don't just go to a healer one day and get healed and that's it. Getting healed, made whole, is a process of becoming yourself. The job of the healer is to facilitate a point of stillness, where your mind stops the chatter, and you get a sense of fully inhabiting your skin. When you're fully inhabiting your skin, nothing else can get in so there'll be no room for disease or illness, because you'll be there instead. Every time you experience this still point, you are deepening in your process of becoming fully who you are. Being who you are in your fullness is what occurs every time you experience the reality of your three tantiens and your spirit body, at which point your consciousness is concentrated in your upper tantien, the cave of original spirit in the centre of your brain. Every time this occurs, you have an opportunity to heal your pains and ailments, by directing chi to the troubled spot. For it is the chi that heals you, and that is what every healer manipulates to effect a cure. Chi is the magic medicine which you release with your mind and has the power to knit broken bones and even rid your body of cancer, as long as you want to be well.

The most consistently effective way of manipulating chi is through the combination of acupuncture and manual chi-transferring, practised by Taoist healers such as this barefoot doctor. Though every attention is paid to alleviating symptoms, it is not the disease itself which is treated, but the person for, no matter what form the disease takes, it is fundamentally merely an expression of dis-ease at the core, which is causing chi to get blocked. When conscious contact is re-established with the core, any deficiency of ease there will vanish. Once the core has eased up, relaxation will radiate outward to the body's surface, enabling the blocked chi to flow freely again and, in time, the symptoms will clear up. If, however, the moment has come to leave your body behind, the facilitation of stillness at the core, during a healing session will ease your passage and help you find tranquillity in the midst of the transition.

You take responsibility for both your condition and your healing. The healer merely helps you heal yourself.

Rather than get involved with orthodox medicine, except where absolutely essential, visit a healer instead. It's not so much the technique being practised that's important, it's the person practising it. No matter whether it's aromatherapy, reiki, shiatsu, massage, acupuncture, cranio-sacral therapy, homeopathy. crystal healing, hypnotherapy, psychotherapy or even good old trepanning (drilling a hole in your scalp), an authentic healer (and you can smell the real thing) will be able to heal you whatever the discipline they practise. The point is, it's you, not them, who heals you, they merely assist you in remembering how.

Visualise the elixir of life, like a rich golden fluid, circulating in your brain, filling every cell, flowing down through your neck, into your chest and abdomen, circulating in your vital organs, down through your hips, circulating in your sexual organs, down through your legs to your feet and your arms to your hands. This rich golden fluid of life, bathing every living cell in your body, is making you new and making you well. Feel new. Feel well.

iNSANiTY
As one nutter to another . . .

Insanity may be like no longer having any control of your computer. No matter which key you press, your hard disc will throw up information at random, not necessarily in any discernible pattern, though often comprising a loop or complex of loops, which cannot easily be turned off.

Insanity lurks beneath the surface of the apparent stability of your consciousness in the dark realms of chaos and flicks you on the ear every time you escape the present moment.

If, as a little youth, when you were too young to have developed a sound psychic structure, you were forced to escape the present moment often because the pain inflicted on you by others was too great and went on for too long for your soul to bear, you may have a propensity for going a little insane from time to time.

But as the world we inhabit is itself completely insane and everyone in it is, to some extent, a lunatic – warders and inmates alike – who's to say who's mad? Insanity is a spiritual journey into the realms of chaos and, wherever possible, those who go there must be treated with the respect due all intrepid explorers. This does not mean, however, that you should confuse respect with stupidity and let some loony with violent tendencies loose in your house.

In the light of the combined madness of the global loony-bin, the only valid criterion for judging insanity is when someone relinquishes their socialising function to the extent that they become a liability for others, and hence a pain in the ass. Up until that point, you can be as mad as a hatter but as long as you keep up your socialising functions, enabling you to continue your dialogue with the outside world coherently enough to get what you need from others and do your bit in return, you'll get away with it. But as soon as you let go of the responsibility for keeping yourself together in the world, and go around raving, chatting fuckrie and making a nuisance of yourself, and keep it up for long enough, they'll come and take you away and stuff you full of chlorpromazine every day till your lips get caked and cracked and your eyes and spirit grow dull enough for them to feel safe to toss you back into the community.

If you feel a madness coming on, go and visit a powerful healer to help you get back in your body and out of the loops in your mind.

Practising the meditations and contemplations in this Handbook over a period of time will help you establish a strong enough psychic structure to accommodate whatever insanity lurks beneath the surface without needing to relinquish your power to others, ie, preserve your fully functional warrior status.

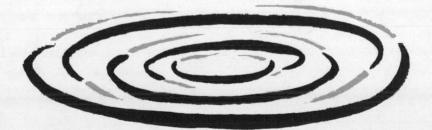

ViOLENCE
Violating the free space of another living being in any way, physically, emotionally and psychically, is a symptom of insanity, unless in self-defence, in which case inflict the minimum damage possible to neutralise your assailant's force and prevent further trouble.

In overcoming your opponent, let your counterattack be devastatingly effective and do not gloat in victory. In being overcome by your opponent, do everything within your power to minimise impact [see *Yielding and Sticking* p. 93], and do not wallow in defeat.

Violence, whether as a one-to-one situation (as in rape, beating, glassing, cutting, clubbing, stabbing, torturing, or murder) or as a group activity (as in gang rape/beating, gang war, civil war, international war and world war) causes huge, ugly, jagged distortions in the energy fields of perpetrators and victims alike, not to mention those of the families and friends of both. These distortions radiate outwards, exponentially, eventually affecting every living being on the planet.

In time these distorted energy patterns complete an entire loop and return to zap the perpetrator with threefold strength (or so the story goes).

So if you want to live in peace yourself, leave others to live in peace. Do everything in your power to prevent or reduce violence wherever you can, and avoid perpetrating it yourself, whether physically, emotionally or psychically. When you are in touch with your true nature – which is essentially comprised of pure, Divine love – it will be cause for deep reflection and offering of prayers to the spirit of your vanquished foe, every time you kill even a mosquito. To actually take the life of another person, except in the most extreme cases of genuine self-defence, is totally out of the question.

Breathe in and out through an imaginary opening in the centre of your chest, and feel peace in your heart. Visualise this peace radiating outwards from your chest, like a fine rose-tinted mist which covers the face of the Earth and neutralises every violent impulse.

Do this every time you feel overwhelmed by despair at the thought of all the violence in the world.

GENEROSiTY
Give, you mean bastard!

Generosity is the art of generating the new in your life, by unconditionally giving away love, chi, information, time, space, money, food or other assorted possessions, as if from an inexhaustible well of abundance, to those you encounter who are temporarily suffering from a deficiency.

Playing this part of the benefactor with an open heart centre requires you adopt the courage to trust that there is an unlimited abundance of whatever's required in the moment, and the belief [see *Belief* p. 87], that whatever you give freely to your world, in the shape of another person/s, will come back to you multiplied; though often not through that same person, or in the same form as it was given.

Give others what they need, and other others will give you what you need. Someone needs 50p (75c) towards a cup of tea or coffee. You give them 50p. You need £50,000 ($75,000) towards a creative project. Someone else will give it to you. That's the basic scheme, though it often works out in less simplistic style. Your world is a continuum, with all parts interlinked and connected at the core.

Giving from your heart, in appropriate form [see *Cool* p. 179] to any part of the continuum is the same as giving to the whole. When you give freely to the whole, the Tao will give freely to you in return. And as the Tao has far more to freely give you than vice versa, you'll be on to a winner.

All things, from the most spiritual substances to the most concrete objects, have their origins in the Tao. The supply at source is inexhaustible. The more you give away of it, the more it creates.

Being the benefactor also requires you open yourself to receive, otherwise the flow will be blocked. Both generosity and receptivity arise from keeping your heart centre open and relaxed.

Visualise an opening in the centre of your chest, through which you're breathing gently in and out. Every inhalation brings the essence of abundance (everything you need) into your life. Every exhalation sends the essence of abundance to those in need.

And say, 'I am living in an abundant world. There is an abundance of all that's necessary in the moment. The more I freely give it away, the more it creates.'

Then simply do abundance (a bun dance)!

MONEY
Money grows on trees.

Money is merely a form of energy/chi. A measure of money equates to a measure of chi.

There is nothing intrinsically wrong or right about money. It is merely an energy measuring device, hence why it's called currency, ie, current, literally that which runs/flows (like water).

Money flows through global society like chi flows through your body. The body parts that are most relaxed, ie, happy and receptive will attract the most chi, the parts that are constricted and depressed will attract the least. But just like this chi balance in the body can be shifted with intention, so also can the balance of money in your life and in global society in general be adjusted by intention. (Money market manipulators do this every day on a global scale.) Money is not the root of all evil. It cannot be, it's only an idea we've all agreed to believe in. It has no intrinsic value of its own. It's a myth. Money is merely a harmless measuring device we use to expedite energy exchange between individuals and groups, which otherwise would become too unwieldy to manage, owing to the high numbers of people interacting.

Greed is the root of all evil.

Greed arises from the mistaken belief or fear that there exists a fundamental shortage of energy/chi, the limited supply of which is depleted every time you give it away. Hence, for you to gain, someone else has to lose. Whereas, in reality, the more energy/chi you use, the more you generate. In basic terms, the more money you have, the more you'll be circulating.

Chi/energy is a spiritual force. Money as a symbol of chi is therefore, by extension, also a spiritual force. Spiritual force is life-enhancing and good, therefore money is good. QED.

The more good, life-enhancing spiritual force (money/wealth) you generate and circulate, the better. Obviously this only applies to money generated by virtuous means which precludes all monies received from violating another person in any way, by dishonesty such as robbery, fraud and deception, whether accompanied by use of physical force or not.

Spend money freely but don't spunk it willy nilly. Contain it like you contain your chi. Spend it with focused intention to get the things you need, just as you do your chi. Don't be stingy as this merely blocks the flow of life for yourself and others.

Whenever you spend money, see it going out from you, doing the rounds of global society and returning to you multiplied.

Every time you spend a penny, say, 'Every penny I spend returns to me multiplied by nine.'

What follows is the money tree visualisation. Perform it at least once a week, and you'll never go short. Two to three days later, there will usually be a noticeable increase in the volume of money coming your way.

Picture yourself sitting under a large, friendly tree, leaning up against its sturdy trunk. Looking up at its many branches, you notice the leaves are actually banknotes of the highest denomination (£50s/$100s). As you sit watching, these notes start falling from the branches and landing all around you on the ground. The more you watch, the faster they fall. As one leaf falls, another one shoots through to replace it. When the notes on the ground around you have formed a big enough pile to fulfil all your current needs (as big or small as you like), gather them up, put them in your pockets/suitcase/truck, etc, say thank you to the money tree, and come back, knowing you can return as often as you choose.

POSSESSIONS
In reality you do not possess anything, not even your body. Everything is on loan, so don't invest chi in hanging on to things. The Tao giveth, and the Tao taketh away. Accept this graciously. You are merely a caretaker.

Keep your chattels to a minimum. Possessions, beyond what you actually need, only drain your chi.

Treading lightly as a warrior means being prepared to let go freely of your possessions at a moment's notice if required by the situation to do so, as in muggings/earthquakes/ariel bombardment by hostile forces/flooding from sudden rises in sea levels/death, etc.

On the other hand, value whatever you have and caretake it to the best of your ability, so that when it passes to someone else, it does so with good chi.

Visualise all your possessions, your houses, clothes, sea-going yachts, jewellery, pots and pans etc, suffused with an electric blue special-effects light, which you're emitting from your cave of original spirit, in centre brain. Picture them glowing with this light, as if they've taken on a life of their own. This helps prevent unconscious chi drainage, makes you get rid of things you no longer need, and magnetises new things that you do need.

RiSK

Always be willing to risk everything you have to keep the story moving on.

Whenever you risk following the spontaneous urges of your heart [see *Spontaneity* p. 102], even if your moves are misjudged, the Tao will always see you right. New opportunities will only come to you when you take risks. This doesn't mean you should risk your life or the lives of others by being impetuous [see *Cool* p. 179].

Say, 'I am willing to risk all I have in order to fulfil my life story.'

ViRTUE

To be an excellent warrior, you have to have virtue. This is not an unattainable idea.

Being virtuous simply means bringing your full authentic self [see *Authorship* p. 81] to bear on the situation you currently find yourself in. It's a moment-by-moment thing, not a permanent state once attained never lost. You fall in and out of the state of virtue as often as you fall in and out of bed.

To achieve it you must be fully centred in your body and fully connected to your imperishable core. This allows your true (spiritual) nature to come through and take over in all your thoughts, words and deeds. When this happens, all your doings will be virtuous. It has nothing to do with morals [see *Amorality vs Morality* p. 106].

AGREEMENTS
Never make a threat or a promise you're not willing to carry out (better not to make them).

When you make an agreement stick to it. Don't use your words idly.

Avoid making any agreements, contracts or commitments, formal or otherwise, with anyone, which you don't feel sure about being able to honour. This applies as much to an informal arrangement to meet your friend at eight as it does to signing a marriage contract. It's always OK to say you don't know, until you're sure one way or the other, or are forced to take a position, in which case you'll know quick enough.

Obviously you are always free to change your mind but when you do, you must be sure to inform everyone involved, so the situation can be fairly renegotiated, and also be willing to accept full responsibility for the consequences.

Every time you goof out on an agreement, however insignificant it seems at the time, you're weakening your link with the universal machinery, which causes obstructions in the flow of energy/chi between you and the world, resulting in poor manifesting ability [see *Manifestation* p.125].

When this occurs, as inevitably it will from time to time (all humans are fallible), don't judge yourself harshly, simply observe [see *Observation vs Judgement* p. 71] with a view to strengthening your resolve to stick to your

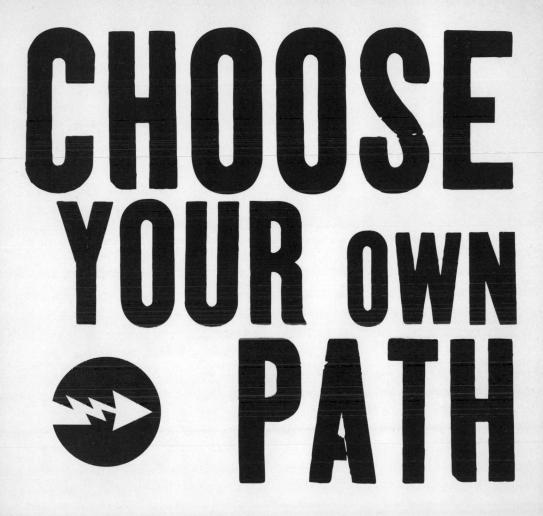

word in future. Additionally, scoop some loop to rebalance your relationship with the universe.

MANNERS
Always be polite, respect all life as your own, and observe the correct protocol.

There is a natural protocol/Tao to every situation, which can only be clearly discerned when your mind is quiet and receptive enough to intuit it and then find the correct, most respectful way to proceed.

Approach everyone you meet as a beloved member of your family. This doesn't mean you must approve of them, or even like them. It simply means you treat them with the respect and kindness you would your own mother or yourself, no matter how scummy they appear.

Everyone you meet has a message or gift for you. Treat everyone as if they were a guru, come to teach you about yourself.

Always establish eye contact, as this creates a link between spirits, which allows the necessary respect, ie, literally seeing afresh, to flow between you. However, beware of getting caught up in the hypnotic stares of those who would take advantage of you [see *Intuition* p. 144].

What starts the fights is when one person feels they are not being seen and therefore not respected by the other. It only takes a split second for this to occur (as in 'road rage'), so care must be taken to stay mindful of what's going on around you. Let others go first, without being a lemon about it, even let others be right, what's important is you remain polite. To do otherwise is so uncool [see *Cool* p. 179] .

COUPLES

it is possible to be both simultaneously a warrior and part of a loving couple that don't drive each other completely mad; i know a few myself. But you'd better be a total master if you want it to last.

To take on the couple scenario, and remain true to yourself as a warrior, with all that implies, requires you both be nothing less than enlightened masters/mistresses.

As this is rarely the case, most couple scenarios end in numbness or tears. People come together unwittingly, to mirror each other, hence to help each other transform, to learn more about themselves and to grow. This does not always take place in the most nurturing, calm or pleasant of ways, and is often painful. We run to relationships to escape our pain, and end up running into it full-on.

After the first three months' flush, when the demons start to surface, and unworkable differences become apparent, you'll inevitably find yourself needing all the powers of clear communication ability at your disposal to negotiate your way with each other. In the ensuing friction, restlessness, dreams of escape and terrors of abandonment you will find the learning.

In the course of all this brouhaha, genuine love may develop and surface between the wintry moments of discontent which, after all, is what you were looking for, and which makes it so damn hard to let go when the end comes (either by death or desertion).

Meanwhile we keep on looking and dreaming.

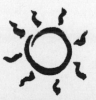

CHILDREN
Children come to us in a state of purity and perfection from the great undifferentiated absolute and then, like everything else on this planet, we fuck them up.

If it's not the mother, it's the father, the babysitter, siblings, teachers, media etc., no one can escape it. Fucked up is the human condition. And well it is, for it is these very distortions arising from the pain of childhood which lend us the colour that makes us interesting for everyone else.

Every little youth that comes through the chute arrives complete with the entire universal blueprint, ready to teach us all.

To abuse a child purposely, physically, emotionally or psychically, even in the slightest way, is a crime against the universe itself, and will set you and probably them back many lifetimes.

Conversely, to save a child from abuse, to rescue a child from the hell of alienation, is to do the universe the greatest of services, and you'll be riding the backs of golden dragons on the winds of the nine celestial heavens for as many eternities as you fancy.

With every new little youth that comes through, also comes the chance for complete redemption of the human race. Always do what you can to protect, preserve and nurture new life.

TAKING POSITIONS
Only take a position when you finally have to, and not a moment before.

Other people will often be pressurising you to make up your mind about this or that. Do not, however, forego your flexibility by assuming a position, until you have no other choice. Remember opinions, ie, positions, are only opinions, which are as changeable as the wind in spring. Respect them, in self and others, but don't take them too seriously.

In fact, don't take anything too seriously and always retain your sense of humour. As a warrior facing the rigours of the challenge, your sense of H is one of your most essential assets, if you want to get to the other side without losing your sanity altogether.

If you think for a moment that the Tao, the gods, goddesses, angels, lesser deities, or whatever, seriously spiritual beings all, aren't sitting there laughing their crown chakras off even as you read this, you're horribly mistaken. The Tao's only in it for the crack [see *Taoism and the Tao* p. 8].

The Tao is able to laugh because it can see all sides, being everywhere and all. This would be impossible had it planted itself resolutely in a fixed position. Be like the Tao. Be flexible. Be fluid.

Keep your mind open to all possibilities until you have no choice but to make a choice, at which point you'll know exactly what to do. Until then, have a laugh.

CHANGE
Everything is in transition. Nothing is permanent except this.

Change is a force you have to groove with, not resist. Like a fast and furious monster of epic proportions, it charges headlong into the deep unknown with you clinging on to its back.

You can't get off, because it's going too fast. It can't stop because constant movement is all it knows.

Though its course is cyclic, you never seem to get back to the same place twice. The story of your life keeps unfolding and there's nothing you can do about it, so you may as well surrender now. Give yourself up to the ride and, with the belief that all things work together for the good, say:

'All change is good. All change is good. All change is good. All change is good. All change is good. All change is good. All change is good. All change is good. All change is good.'

Good!

TiME MANAGEMENT
Time is endless.

Though it's also passing by at sixty minutes per hour, so if you find yourself with much to achieve, it's best to divide it up into chunks, into which you can pre-fit the tasks before you.

Once having visualised yourself successfully completing your load within the allotted slot, when the moment actually arrives you then have the choice to stretch or shrink it depending on how dull or exciting the project is.

The speed of passing of a chunk of time is relative to how interested or bored you are with what you're doing. It is perfectly possible, therefore, to effectively stretch time in order to get superhumanly warrior-like amounts done.

Conversely, you can shrink it when you're bored, such as during a dull class at school or an endless long-haul flight. It is best not to shrink it too much, though, because it's your life you're rushing through.

Develop a strong working partnership with an appointment book or organiser, and be disciplined about allotting realistic portions of time to each upcoming activity. Be firm, though not obsessive, about staying with the plan, but always remain mentally flexible enough to move with the unexpected. Make use of lists and diagrammatic illustrations to organise your thoughts, but avoid using list preparation as a procrastinatory device.

Be punctual. Being late is a power ploy and is tantamount to stealing other people's time. Being early is not really a problem as long as you don't peak too soon and burn out.

If you are habitually late, work with this affirmation:

'It is impossible for me to be late for anything. Nothing can start for me till I get there.'

To stretch time, simply state at the start of the particular time slot you wish to stretch, talking directly to your own spirit body: 'Stretch this time!'

(I'm not going to tell you how to shrink it! What you rushing for anyways?)

TRANSMUTiNG POLLUTANTS
Embrace filth.

If you base your faith on the theory that whatever is, is whatever's meant to be and that everything works together for the good, then all that vast, stinking, insidious mess of pollution in our air, water, food and sunlight must be there to help you mutate along the lines evolution always intended for you.

Don't resist the pollution, welcome it in as a catalyst for evolutionary change. Transmute it into chi with the power of your intention. Trust your chi, slightly soiled though it may be, to protect you and continue down the Great Thoroughfare without a second glance.

If it turns out you were wrong to have harboured this belief, at least you won't have wasted years walking around like a sad environment-victim [see *Authorship* p. 81, *Self-Pity* p. 110 and *End-of-the-World Phobia* p. 119].

Say, 'I have the power to transmute all poison into positive life-enhancing chi.' You may need to repeat this no less than sixty-three times for it to penetrate to the deeper layers of your circuitry.

MEDiA POLLUTiON

Everything you see on TV/the movies, download off the net, hear on radio and CDs, or read in newspapers, magazines and books, including this Handbook, is someone else's idea.

As with all ideas, a small proportion of the countless squillions dumped on your hard disk everyday, are useful.

The major portion, however, are best dragged directly into the trash.

What you see on TV as news is, in fact, only a version of the event. That version has been influenced by so many spurious, subjective factors, including commercial and political considerations, that it cannot be blindly accepted as 'the truth'.

In the course of the day, what with all the billboards, advertising slogans on passing sweatshirts and trainers, messages on rear windscreens, and sound snippets from doors that open and close as you walk by, as well as your usual 'chosen' media intake, your senses are mugged and your spirit raped to the quick with other people's thoughts.

There is nothing you can do about this, other than to ease off from that TV, etc, but if you remain aware of the media pollution going on around you; it tends to diffuse its power over you.

Additionally, if you consciously welcome in this mental poison, you can transmute it by the power of your intention, into pure intelligence, by simply stating to yourself:

'I am automatically transmuting all media pollution into pure intelligence. My mind uses all incoming information to enrich me.'

As well as being a punter/consumer of other people's ideas, contribute some of your own whenever possible. Broadcast your own unique message of salvation to the world, through every medium available to you. Don't be shy. We've got the channels, but we're still a bit lacking in content.

And we want information. Who knows, yours may be the message we've all been waiting for.

GOODBYES ARE SUCH A FUCK!

People come into your orbit. People go out of your orbit. in, out. in, out. it's the basic yin-yang, contraction-expansion motion of the ocean of existence itself.

It's so hard to say, 'goodbye, farewell, may your road be gentle and take you to beautiful places, and may your life be positively affected in great measures of ten thousand increments each from reading this Handbook', but that time has finally come. It's hard on account of my separation anxiety.

I've become attached to you. I've been sitting for what seems like so long now, writing to you, presumptuously reaching for contact with the deepest part of your person, that I've grown to love you. And I don't even know what you look like.

I've been writing to you from my creative confinement in various huts and bungalows all over Southern Thailand, hotel rooms in the Balearics, and secret locations in London (metropolis of cool).

It's been a long, varied and challenging labour, but the baby's out now, and I'd like to thank you sincerely for reading it.

(You're a bona fide warrior now! Send off for your membership card and secret siren ring.)

Obviously there's loads I must have left out, and much more to say besides, but there's more coming down the shoot (watch out).

Later.

Barefoot Doctor

ACKNOWLEDGEMENTS

I wish to acknowledge my gratitude to everyone who has helped me with this project, and specifically:

Jane Hajioff, (Agent Jane), whose support went ten thousand measures of distance beyond the call of duty, and without whom the writing process would have been a lot lonelier than it was.

Queen Beanie Venturini, for the non-warrior Valentino shirt, which threw the urban warrior into such strong definition.

Joe Russell, whose undying support over the years and as-it-went-along manuscript approval and youth-culture ratification kept me going through the dark.

Jake Russell for being a hero, and giving me pure, fresh strength when mine was flagging.

Michael Angelo Russell, transatlantic star, for your shining visits.

Niel Spencer, don of the dons, for original media ratification of Barefoot Doctor entity, and say-so for the Handbook.

Paul Bradshaw, for providing cultural milieu.

Kath Willgress, for original ratification of writer status.

Paul Tulley, for Hoxton Square Tulleyman buzz.

Kathy Acker, for ratification of author status.

Liz Russell and Claire Amerena for raising the boys and giving BFD space to make a noise.

David, Jonathan, Susan, Nicola, Vicci, Colin, Victoria, et al for the warmth and light of Spirit.

Grum The Baptist-Antony Somers, for the full-contact brawls, warrior inspiration and being such a brother.

Vanessa Kramer, for Lebensraum and Gemütlichkeit (home comforts).

Sam Kramer, for being such an honest rogue and sharing a home.

The late Frank B Kramer, for continued support and guidance from the other side (can you read this?).

The late R D Laing, for the odd howl from the other side.

Mina Symeon, for not fearing the depths of the abyss.

Jo Simons, for continual support, love and adolescent madness.

Arun Kumar, undercover holy man, for many healings in the Grove and various media maraudings.

David, the big H, Herman, for the unstoppable force.

Michelle Ziff, for the kitchen Lakshmi connection.

Adam Simmonds, for many late night printing sessions and being such a giezer.

Shirley, The Girlie, (my mum) for original template and support from the start of the overall project (ie, me).

Victor, The Victor, (my dad), for that original thrust.

Stewart Imber, for life-saving and providing the firm but gentle voice of reason over the years.

Stevo Nakovitch, for being there the whole time with undying assistance and support.

Sonny Spruce, for first injection of authentic cool.

Patria C Barbary, for unconditional God-Mother love.

Scott MacHardy, for mountain lore.

Katie MacHardy, for keeping Scott together.

Rowan O'Neal, for being such a courageous witch.

Vivianne Thompson (Spider Woman), for keepin' the Taos home fires burning.

Bob Jacobs, for the sacred pipe.

Craig, Le Baron, Newman, (and, of course, the Baroness), for continued support, business maraudings, and being so suave.

Zoé Redman, for original ratification of artist status and after-book personal restoration.

Nemo Jones, for consistent creative inspiration, sublime music and brotherley support, giezer.

Jonty Champelovier, for introducing me to the grand design.

Jack Pollit, for brotherly support and major urban re-education programme.

Darcy Mathews, for helping me through the midway crisis.

Anna Bluman, for simply being so damn beautiful.

Alex Fuller, for exemplary urban warrior-like inspiration.

Yehudi Gordon, for getting me started and taking me back into the fold.

Janet Balakas, for original push into the author business.

Richard Taffler, for boldly continuing to be the Professor.

David Freeman, for helping me not take positions.

Ailon Free, for staying free.

Jessica Brown, for continued love and support and San Francisco linkage.

Harriet, for such elegant encouragement.

Mary Queen of Scotts, Minaxe Patel, and all that tribe of fierce London women, for not having me run out of town. All my friends, students and patients, for believing in me.

Judy Piatkus, for taking such a gracious punt.

Anne Lawrance, for being the kindest and most considerate commissioning editor.

Finally, my own Self, for being so thoroughly cooperative and pleasant to work with throughout this project, cheers!

iNDEX

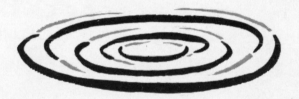